THE WAY THEY HEALED

From the Egyptians to the Essenians

AN APPROACH TO THE THERAPY
Understanding and Practicing

DANIEL MEUROIS

THE WAY THEY HEALED

From the Egyptians to the Essenians

AN APPROACH TO THE THERAPY
Understanding and Practicing

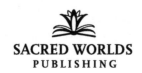

SACRED WORLDS
PUBLISHING

The Way They Healed: From the Egyptians to the Essenians. An Approach to the Therapy: Understanding and Practicing

Original French title:
Ainsi Soignaient-ils … des Egyptiens aux Esséniens, une approche de la thérapie: comprendre et pratiquer

© 2003 Éditions Le Perséa, Montréal – © 2008 Le Passe-Monde
Author: Daniel Meurois

© 2021 Sacred Worlds Publishing for the English edition
www.sacredworldspublishing.com

The moral rights of the author have been asserted.

Translated by: Isabelle Laak
Editing: Catherine Hensley
Cover Art: SoulfulBrand | soulfulbrand.com
Book Production: WildGraphics | asawild.org

2021 ISBN: 978-0-9987417-3-4

To Marie Johanne,
for her healing hands and her so vivid memory ...

Table of Contents

ALSO BY

Introduction

I hesitated for a long time before I started writing this book. After the publication of *Les Robes de Lumière*[1] a few years ago, I thought I had finished my personal participation with a wide audience, a different approach to disease and therapy. How to read the aura, the subtle bodies, was the central point of *Les Robes de Lumière*.

Obviously, since then[2] things have evolved enormously. Much research has been done, and many doors have been opened both collectively and individually.

In this vast movement of reflection and experimentation, I have naturally been much more deeply involved in investigating the energy field and how it is structured in the human body.

Over the years, my perceptions have become more precise. As the information flowed, I found myself with new knowledge coming constantly to nourish another approach to this equilibrium we call "health."

However, I felt bound to limit the spread of this information to a small number of relatives because my research was being carried out at a time of great interest in the so-called "alternative therapies," which was leading to more therapists than sick persons! I didn't want to feed what was becoming a trend.

---

1 *Les Robes de Lumière (The Robes of Light) by Anne and Daniel Meurois-Givaudan, 2011. First published in 1987 by Editions Amrita (France).*

2 *1987.*

My position has changed today[3] because it seems to me that we have fortunately gone to another level—that of a sorting, a digestion of information, and, consequently, a maturation.

As a result, true therapists have emerged, able to accompany human beings in the depths of their overall health.

When I say "true therapists," I am referring to those who practice or learn—often both at once—apart from any controlling power or fundamentalism but with competence, honesty, passion, and compassion.

I finally decided to write these pages for them, and also for all those I gladly call the "sincere apprentices of life." These people, without calling themselves therapists, aspire to know a little more about themselves while seeking to do, modestly, as much good as possible around them. They are the most numerous, and the reason for the review of certain basic notions in this text.

The book I am presenting to you here is certainly a workbook, a book about a method, but also and above all a book about an attitude of the heart and soul. In this sense, it can be addressed to any human being whose wish is simply to grow by approaching a little better the amazing marriage of the subtle energy and the dense matter in each person.

Where does my information come from? From the same source of my previous books. It comes from my natural ability to cross the boundaries of the worlds, a capacity that has only increased with the integration of a major finding—that we are primarily vibrational beings. This vibrational nature of our reality clearly operates simultaneously on several levels of existence, which constantly interfere with each other. This also means that the subtle already exists in the dense and that the line that separates them has an extraordinary porosity.

To turn toward the whole health of the being and to try to maintain it in balance, one must constantly have in

---

3   *"Today" here is sometime in 2002, as this book was first published in 2003.*

mind the sense of its unity through the perception of its multidimensionality. It is in this direction that I am proposing we go in *The Way They Healed*.

Developing such a vision and integrating it into a therapeutic practice represents, one will agree, the work of a lifetime. As such, this book does not claim to be anything more than an additional milestone in the attempt to comprehensively understand the functioning of the human body.

Its originality, and why I finally wanted to write this book, is undoubtedly due to the fact that it restores as faithfully as possible certain practices that took place around the Mediterranean Basin a few thousand years ago.

I am referring to the Egyptian civilization in the Amarna Period, under Pharaoh Akhenaten, as well as the Essenian therapeutic tradition, which was its direct successor.

It would be very wrong to consider the knowledge from these ancient times as a collection of superstitions just good enough to trigger a smile. Many practices from these epochs coincide in a surprising way with certain elements of so-called "holistic medicine" today.

In light of my investigations into the past and my own experiences, I return once more to this observation: Our current practices are not the result of real discoveries in the primary sense of the term. They are rediscoveries of basic truths relating to the human body. They are rediscoveries of basic truths relating to the human body under other notions of references used in the past. They only resurface nowadays under other grids of references than those used in the past.

I firmly believe that no medicine should exclude another. Wisdom comes from knowing how to handle each intelligently by accepting that all can participate in the development of a coherent ensemble.

It is in this state of mind that I now give you the following method of work in this book—not by seeking to create or nurture another school but in the hope of expanding the field of the human mind while providing your hands and heart with some additional tools.

Good thinking, and good practice!

Part One

Chapter I

A Sacred Gaze

1) Once Upon a Time ...

In the course of my many investigations into what is today known as the "Akashic library,"[1] I had the opportunity to very regularly spend time in therapy centers.

Whether in Egypt at the time of Akhenaten or in Palestine's Essenian communities, what's always struck me is that these centers were far from being only simple hospitals or clinics.

In those times that seem to us more distant than they actually are, the notions of health and illness were necessarily linked to the sacred dimension of the human being.

The body was not considered an improved earthy mechanism. They first perceived it as a tangible part of the whole, its roots in an immeasurable celestial universe, the universe of the Divine.

The physical body—the palpable—was thus approached as the final link in the chain of creation. The dense matter represented the first bar of the ladder by which a human could go back to the subtle Ocean of Causes.

---

1   *Akashic Records.*

Any therapist or master of this art knew that he had to climb as high as possible along this ladder to identify one origin or more of a disease, and then try to deactivate it.

Since a human being was perceived as a kind of tree with primarily celestial roots, his inner balance could not be compromised. That's why most health centers were also temples. Everything was ordered around the sacred dimension of the being. It was not unusual for a center to be called a "House of Life" and considered a place of initiation—that is, a place of passage in every sense of the term. One could not, therefore, be a therapist without also being a priest, or without having devoted enough time to authentic, metaphysical reflection.

Such training naturally resulted in a higher awareness, which meant that death was no longer perceived as being in opposition to life, nor sickness to health. Health, sickness, and death were seen as the different stages of metamorphosis of a great current of life in perpetual motion. The multiple manifestations of these stages lead only to a great and sublime purpose: the maturation of human consciousness and its purification in preparation for blissfulness to come. Thus, it was taught that, contrary to appearances, nothing was opposed to anything. Death did not cry out in defeat of life, and disease simply translated a lack of harmonious dialogue between the soul and the body.

Starting from these certainties, the different schools of therapists always tried to teach in a way that took into account the eminently sacred character of the Ocean of Life we live in, which crosses us at every moment.

It is certainly not my intention to plead here for the restoration of such a system of priests, temples, and therapies. While it had its greatness and beauty, it also produced its share of excesses and aberrations. I mention it here to draw attention to the dryness and desacralized nature of our modern-day health care systems.

Which hospital or clinic can honestly claim to be a place of health today? How many doctors or practitioners feel they happily go to work each morning to a place that exudes hope for healing? A tiny quantity, no doubt.

Finally, what sick person can let go enough to talk about her soul to a technician at the controls of a machine[2] that will "cut" her body into slices?

My purpose is to simply take what was good from the past and teach it to us now—namely, the vision of who we are and the search for a setting where beauty and kindness also play their healing roles.

2) Preliminary Conditions

a) The Sanctuary

Let's dare to use this expression: "Create a sanctuary." This sanctuary will not be linked to any dogma; instead, it will be a sanctuary of all possibilities, a place of tender light and freedom. Because that's what must exist for a place to participate in the restoration of harmony between body and soul.

Your therapy room will be a place in which you feel deeply at home, a place with the colors of your soul, of course, but also neutral enough to match the nuances of the heart of all those who will enter.

According to Egyptian and Essenian rules, the ideal is to maintain a certain sobriety in the room. All objects, utilitarian or symbolic, will be chosen according to the purity of their aesthetics. It is important to understand that these objects will become in many ways bridges, or reference points—in other words, connections a patient will rediscover with happiness at each visit.

Let us not forget that a symbol is a living presence connected to an archetype and that a judiciously placed light can promote the state of consciousness attached to it. In the same way, a well-chosen a resin incense burner, for example, will facilitate the resonance of the being with what she is

---

2   *An MRI scan.*

receiving. You will understand without difficulty that both the therapist and the client receiving the treatment are greatly influenced by how the sanctuary is set up.

A real sanctuary suggests a space out of time, parentheses allowing an intimate dialogue that is horizontal as well as vertical. The human being is called to be in communion with the Divine, not only in a receptive but also an emissive way.

When the beauty of a sanctuary or healing room is simple, suggesting the idea of a bridge, it will be easier for the therapist and the client to connect to the multiple levels of their multidimensionality. Let us remember that beauty does not only mean pleasure for the eye. It is first and foremost a caress for the soul, an elixir that makes her gently open.

b) Ritual of the Solstices

All the great traditions agree on this point: There is no real sanctuary without the consecration of it. But what exactly is a consecration? It is a natural gesture, an offering. It is an offering of what goes beyond us, of what passes through us and drives us to love. It is an absolute dedication to life.

In this sense, there is no need to refer to a particular faith to consecrate a place and then trace the sacred perimeter of it. As the human heart is a perfect point of marriage between what is known as Above and Below, all that is required for the consecration to become effective is simply that the therapist be pure, loving, and happy.

Pharaoh Akhenaten believed that the true priesthood state was in fact a state of mastery—a mastery in the alignment of our different worlds, something any human being can accomplish outside of a religious context, and one which he spontaneously experienced during privileged moments.

It is in such a state of mind, open and nondogmatic, that I communicate to you this very simple ritual that was developed at the end of Akhenaten's reign and subsequently used for the consecration of the Essenian "bethsaids," or wellness centers.

It was repeated twice a year, that is to say at each of the two solstices. It was an opportunity for the therapist to renew his covenant of love or his alliance with the Divine while ensuring the purification of his healing room.

How to Proceed:

- A day before a solstice, place good pinches of sea salt in the corners of your treatment room. This salt will aspirate, absorb, and dissolve the eventual residual energies of the ethereal dimensions of your room.

- On the solstice day, with the help of good incense (the therapeutic incense of the Tibetan tradition, for instance) or a small bag of dry sage, walk around your room in a clockwise direction three times.

- Then repeat this walk with a feather in your hand. With the help of this feather, you will trace signs in the air. The Egyptians and Essenians used the Ankh cross, today called the Cross of Egyptian Life, a symbol of fertility and balance. You can, however, use the Christian cross if you prefer or any other great symbol closer to your personal preference. The idea is to lower the energy footprint in the etheric counterpart of your treatment room. With its constitution, the feather has always been recognized as a powerful sensor of subtle energy. That's why, ideally, it is desirable that you find one that is a pretty good size. (A goose feather will work well.) The next step of your consecration is to light a flame in the center of your room. In the past, this was done with an oil or camphor lamp, but today it is better to use a candle, which is easier to handle.

- Sit down facing this flame. After a moment of personal recentering, quickly pass your hands open over the flame. Then, in the same movement, skim the top of your head with your two palms. This is a back-and-forth movement that you will repeat three times. Its function is to purify the etheric nature of your own aura through a vibrational resonance with the subtle counterpart of the Fire Element. Do not just think of a nice symbol. Perform these gestures in true communion with the Spirit of Fire.

- Now comes the prayer and the invocation. Again, rely on the impulses of your heart and the sensitivity that characterizes you. I would highly recommend the following hymn because of its universal essence. This hymn was created by the college of therapists working directly with Akhenaten.

> *"O You, Sun of the Uncreated,*
> *Bless and consecrate this room,*
> *Not as a place of power,*
> *But as a point of balance,*
> *Of reparation, consolation, and accuracy*
>
> *O You, Sun of the Uncreated,*
> *Live in this body and in this heart,*
> *These hands and this mouth,*
> *Not using the body as a servant*
> *But rather as your perfect temple."*

- The consecration will ideally be concluded with a time of meditation. However, it goes without saying that the whole of this ritual will have to be accomplished in full awareness—that is, with a meditative mind.

- Obviously, such a practice is not a mechanical task that is done just to "do it right." The conscience of the one who consecrates his or her sanctuary has for its mission connecting with the divine source in order to work in symbiosis with the place and what it represents.

c) The Therapist's Clothes

Among the ancients, clothing was of major importance. A garment had to reflect the image of purity with which they wished to work. Clothing helped to create this image both for themselves and those they cared for. Like the decoration of their sanctuary of therapy, they saw their clothing as a point of reference or landmark—a mental and emotional point of reference that a client might need along the way to the hoped-for healing.

Of course, we are not adopting such a systematic attitude regarding clothing because times are different nowadays. Everyone knows that the clothes don't make the man. Fortunately, the days of wearing a robe of a certain color in order to be credible are gone.

Still, there is a point to be made on the subject of clothing I consider part of the concept of the landmark important. A truly suffering person lives in a sort of dispersion, whether at the level of their vital forces, the level of their inner being, or on both levels at the same time. Having a stable and unified image of their therapist can be an additional aid to the gathering and focusing they are trying to reclaim.

It is obvious that the quality of a treatment is not systematically conditioned by the visual considerations I'm talking about here. However, the way in which a treatment is received—the conditions of its reception—is a factor that must not be neglected. The image a therapist presents can sometimes, unconsciously, influence the width of the opening of the doors by which their treatment is being welcomed.

When harmony becomes a rallying sign, it ends up multiplying the impact of a technique.

11

To conclude, it seems important to me to add that this is not a matter of making a big "fuss" over some ritual or aesthetic notions of a therapeutic approach.

The ideal is to comply with the advice of this chapter and live the sacred aspect but still remain in a place of solemnity, simplicity, and discretion. These three qualities keep us from taking ourselves too seriously or becoming rigid in some routines. Ultimately, the work becomes inseparable from a real job done with love.

Chapter II

The Alignment of the Therapist

1) Healing: A State of Spirit

Although this book offers a practical therapeutic method and details a number of treatments, it is certainly not meant to be technical in the cold sense of the term.

The exercises will be of little value if they are understood and applied as simple recipes. In truth, they represent only the apparent or emerging part of what will help others. I mean that technicity is only the last wheel of the vehicle that will move us.

Being a therapist is more than simply displaying a diploma or aligning a certain amount of intellectual and mechanical knowledge. This term—"therapist"—connotes a quality of being and a dimension of the heart that have nothing to do with the optional activity of "studying to become a therapist." The student-therapists of Egypt and the Essenian fraternity were not recruited from among those who showed themselves only capable of absorbing knowledge.

They were observed for many months, sometimes years, to ensure their profound humanity and radiance. The ability to listen and charisma were the first traits sought by the teachers tasked with choosing and then training the student-therapists.

Being a therapist is first a state of mind or spirit. I am aware, in writing these words, that such a statement is obvious, but I am also aware, from experience, that it is good to be reminded of those things.

When I talk about a state of spirit, this is beyond the state of the soul—namely, beyond the possible fluctuations of one's moods, emotions, and personal life.

In this approach, *the spirit* to which I'm referring is what the Easterners call *"atma,"* or the absolute diamond of one's Consciousness. It is about the essence of your being, of What it is in you that cannot be soiled or hurt. I'm talking about the most virginal and powerful part of yourself, of what is by nature in close and permanent contact with the Divine Reality.

A therapist's goal is for his sanctuary to be in resonance with this space within the Infinite. With this internal approach, a provided treatment is therefore never "an act of ego" on the part of the therapist

The therapist instead becomes the intermediary between the dimensions of the subtle and the realm of our earthy existence. This means that healing does not belong to him on his own. He does not make it his personal challenge since he is not at war with anything. He does not fight but rather strives to pacify, renew links, and restore the bridges through which vital currents can play their role again.

In understanding the meaning of all this, it's clear that it is the therapist's overall view of himself and life as well that must remain vigilant in the sense of a permanent concern for truth.

On the pediments of some of the Egyptian houses of life, one could read the following inscription: *"We offer what we are."* This meant that transparency was sought first and foremost, and that only the fluidity of being a therapist allowed for the spreading of a certain healing light. On the basis of this, it must be understood that the intensity of a therapeutic session of approaching the human energy field is proportional to the humility, in the noble sense of the term, with which it is given.

In the same way, the mastery of some Essenian therapists resulted from a state of service incompatible with any idea of the domination of a vibration. In fact, true mastery is radically foreign to the concept of domination. Domination uses control and force, whereas mastery leads to a more far-reaching yet intimate comprehension and thus invites you to acquire the altitude necessary to reach the desired goal.

2) Prove?

The idea of having to prove anything should not even occur to a therapist. I recall an anecdote about Master Jesus, who was directly from, as we now know, the Essenian community in Palestine.[1]

He was called to the bedside of a woman suffering for many days with terrible abdominal pain. Asked to intervene, He simply put his hands on her sick belly and then went away. That same evening, He inquired about the health of the woman. He was told by his disciple, "She walks again because all the pain has disappeared. But some say that it is the decoction of plants she drank a little before your arrival that cured her." "So what?" said Master Jesus, his disciple uncomfortable with such an attitude of detachment.

He said again, "So what?" and then in a rather amused tone, "Did not you tell me she was healed? This is enough for me."

This story illustrates quite well on its own a whole level of consciousness that merits consideration. We live today in a society in which everyone is indoctrinated with the notion of having to constantly prove his or her own value, his or her own success. The notion of performance is thus omnipresent, quietly becoming a poison for the soul and the body. It is obviously legitimate, though, for a therapist to work with the

---

1   *The Way of the Essenes: Christ's Hidden Life Remembered by Anne and Daniel Meurois-Givaudan.*

hope of a great result, and it would not make sense for her to get out of the picture while displaying a low profile. False humility is certainly a weakness as well as a pretension.

But this story teaches us about the vanity of a claim. There should be no fighting, nothing in a state of opposition, when it comes to the health of a human being. To a true therapist, it doesn't matter whether it's this method or another that is used to overcome pain. The therapist's satisfaction is first based on the well-being of the client she is treating, even though that client is not "her client." For what concerns us here, there is no honor list to get on!

With the descriptions of this ideal attitude, I invite you to step further into preparation.

3) **Preparatory Exercises:** *Expansion of the Nadis*

The network of "nadis" of the human body is comparable to a blood or nervous network. It is through this network that the life force called *"prana"* irrigates the etheric body: the first subtle body that defines a living being.[2]

Some nadis are similar to rivers, others to streams, and still others to creeks.

With their layout associated with the chakras, the role of the nadis is to frame the structure of the physical body. Its existence is consequently anterior to the body. That's why it's so important for a therapist to maintain his own network of nadis.

The "drive belt" that it represents during a treatment requires that it be maintained in a regular way. The following exercise is analogous to a "dredging" of alluvium in a river. It has the effect of cleaning or even scaling.[3]

---

2   See p. 18, *The Great Book of Essenian & Egyptian Therapies by Daniel Meurois & Marie Johanne Croteau.*

3   *In dentistry, the term "scaling" means tartar removal.*

In the course of its thousand activities, your body produces waste materials, some of which will be housed along your nadis just as fats gradually and excessively deposit on the walls of your arteries if you eat poorly. The waste that concerns the network of nadis is essentially composed of psychic and respiratory debris. Clearly, it is the nature of one's thoughts and the way you breathe that generate it. In other words, the quality and quantity of prana you invite to circulate in your nadis make them properly irrigated or, on the contrary, clogged up. In summary, the expansion of your energy circulation system is crucial if you want to let the prana to play its role as a repairer, builder, and transmitter.

Here's how to proceed after taking the time necessary to become aware of your body as a tree whose roots are deep in the ground. (This awareness is essential for all the exercises that follow.)

Exercise #1

- Seated or standing, invite a Presence of Light, to caress your coronal chakra (seventh chakra).

- Take a short breath in while internally calling for a light point from the top of your head to go down between your two eyes at the level of your sixth chakra. Then breathe out slowly and bring up the light point to the top of your head.

- Start a second breath in, identical to the first, and let the light point go down to your throat at the level of the fifth chakra. Breathe out.

- Continue this exercise with four other inhalations and exhalations to bring your light point to all the chakras until it reaches the base chakra.

Don't forget that each inhaling and exhaling movement must be done gently, without tension, and with a maximum of awareness of the light point that will "brush" you.

In reality, this is more about the inner perception of a luminous presence descending progressively along your vertical axis than a strict visualization. Therefore, it does not come from your imagination but instead the intimate connection of a reality operating in an effective way. Finally, I will specify that it is not necessary to direct the luminous point back to the top of the skull at each expiration. Letting go is preferable.

When the exercise is mastered, you will able to perform it with ease. I recommend practicing it by replacing the luminous point with a column of light, which will do the same work of cleaning from top to bottom.

Ideally, this exercise should be repeated seven times in a row. I am saying ideally because, first of all, it is up to you to respect your own rhythm and not force yourself.

If you can practice it daily, I only recommend doing it once a day. Don't go faster, which could lead to over cleaning and physiological disturbances.

Exercise #2

- After laying your hands, palms up, on your knees, center your consciousness for a few moments in the center of your chest.

- Try to perceive the sun of your heart chakra. Its presence will feel like a spring freshness.

- From the center of this sun, let a luminous spiral unfurl that radiates all over your chest. This spiral, which will eventually be vertical and flattened on the rib cage, will spin out slowly clockwise while you inhale.

- When your lungs are full, exhale slowly, making sure that the spiral is running, or starting to turn in a counterclockwise movement.

You will repeat this cycle ideally eight times in a row.

Like Exercise One, this exercise should be practiced in its entirety only once a day. You can do it in addition to the first exercise or alternate between the two, depending on your interior comfort with both exercises. This comfort is a barometer you must consult periodically.

You cannot settle in with a practice unless you harmonize with it.

If an inconvenience occurs (for example, dizziness or headaches) in the early days, this should not be a concern. These are usually due to the "unlocking" of energy doors caused by the unusual intake of prana in the body. They should disappear by persevering a little and measuring the approach of the exercises.

Exercise #3

The Method of the Master

Here finally is a complete practice in the form of a series of exercises. These were taught by Christ to a small circle of disciples. This is probably the first time in 2,000 years that they have been shared with a wide audience.

This set of exercises is for not only students of the energy therapies but also any person who wishes to undertake a deep cleaning of their network of nadis while harmoniously developing all of their chakras.

Because of the complex and powerful components, I recommend this series for those who have already become familiar with breathing and visualization techniques.

This practice is composed of eight major phases. I strongly recommend progressing to a new phase only after you've fully integrated the previous phase, meaning you have mastered it without experiencing any discomfort.

Master Jesus instructed his disciples to practice one exercise at a time for seven days in a row. The whole series of exercises took up to eight weeks.

At the end of the eight weeks, he trained his disciples to complete the set of exercises in eight days (first day, first exercise; second day, second exercise; and so on).

If one of his disciplines had difficulty putting into practice one of the eight phases (and experienced discomfort, dizziness, etc.), He asked him to momentarily stop the exercise by not forcing anything. Then He advised the disciple to move on to the next exercise, like nothing was wrong, with the goal of not turning the difficulty into a problem.

Master Jesus, however, would guide the disciple to reflect on the area that was creating a discomfort, an emotional reaction, or dizziness. Such a reflection was oriented on the symbolic character of the area in question. It was in no way polemical or dualistic; rather, it was meditative.

A good technician does not necessarily understand better than another the deep essence of what he sets in motion.

Similarly, all masters of meditation know that the exercises they teach are only occasional instruments. These instruments cannot take away the bitterness of a dry heart. Only compassion—the fruit of a soul—is the miracle that can help a therapist reach the "fifth season" (the fifth dimension or 5D consciousness, where one is capable of accessing the higher vibration levels of a being). If we compare one's whole being to a light bulb of the highest and most sophisticated quality, what will this bulb be used for if it is not connected to an adequate source of energy? A broken promise, nothing more.

Here is the whole of this practice as it was taught by Christ. Ideally, each exercise should be done only when one is comfortably installed on the ground.[4]

a) Purification of the First Chakra (Base Chakra)

- Place both hands on your knees, palms down.

- Pay attention to the base of your body, and try to feel roots digging into the ground, just as if you were a tree. Maintain this inner attitude as you try to perceive a kind of gravity, accompanied by the sensation of sinking into the ground, or at least becoming one with it.

- Now bring your attention above your head, and feel the presence of a beautiful ball of white light. Invite it to slowly descend into you until flooding your base chakra.

- Breathe in peacefully through the nose while visualizing the winding of a luminous spiral at the base of your body. Roll out this coil while exhaling. (Note that the arrow in Figure 1 below indicates the direction of this run.)

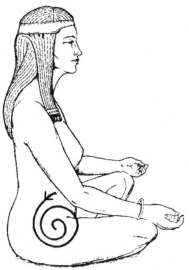

---

4   *The lotus position in yoga.*

Practice seven inhalations/exhalations of this type, breathing freely between each.

b) Purification of the Second Chakra

- Place your left hand on your left knee, palm down, while your right hand is positioned on your second chakra.

- Place your left hand on your left knee, palm down, while your right hand is positioned on your second chakra.

- Let your consciousness descend from your back to the base of your body by perceiving a white sun there. Bring it up to your second chakra with a short breath in.

- Then, bring this sun down to the base chakra with a short breath out.

- Ideally, repeat four sets of seven inhalations/exhalations. Between each set, take care to observe a deep silence and focus your attention on your second chakra.

Note that with each breath in and out, the air should gently scrape the back of the nasal cavity, causing a slight noise.

c) Purification of the Third Chakra

- Place your left hand on your left knee, palm down, while your right hand is positioned on your third chakra.

- With a breath in, visualize that same white sun that descended from your back to the base of your body. Move it to your third plexus and let it sit, shining, for a few seconds.

- Then exhale powerfully, always through your nose, with a sharp blow while trying to perceive a total expansion of your aura.

The ideal scenario is repeating these inhalations/ exhalations thirty-three times. You must be very careful in this practice. When it is understood well, this should not lead to hyperventilation—that is, when it is conducted peacefully and with care. You will end this exercise by observing a long inner silence.

d) Purification of the Fourth Chakra

- Cross your arms over your chest, right over left.[5]

- Sit and breathe regularly, trying to perceive (without projecting forward) a flattened spiral of pink light swirling harmoniously in the center of your chest. Its direction of rotation is clockwise. Ideally, nineteen complete rotational movements will occur, and your breathing will remain at its natural pace.

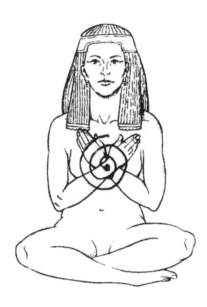

---

5   *Similar to the image of a pharaoh with his arms crossed over his chest, holding the cross of justice in one hand and a whip in the other, forming a full "X" of protection and empowerment.*

- Then have a column of white light rise from your heart chakra to the top of your head, with a slow breath in.

- At the end of your breath in, once the column of light has reached above your head, let it spin and form a spiral turning clockwise. Perceive it while holding your breath briefly.

Ideally, this exercise will be performed four times in a row.

e) Purification of the Fifth Chakra

- Place your left hand on your left knee, palm up, while your right hand is positioned on your throat chakra.

- Slowly and consciously, inhale a trickle of light blue air while scraping the back of your nasal cavity with it.

- Exhale the trickle of air in the same way while visualizing this time a dark blue color. This will be a load of etheric waste.

Practice this respiratory movement seven times in a row to complete the "cleansing" phase of this exercise before beginning the "toning" phase.

- Make a buzzing sound that emanates from the back of your throat. When you approach the end of your breath, finish expelling it at once through the nose with force.

Repeat this phase five times in a row and then remain in a deep silence.

f) Purification of the Sixth Chakra

- After putting your hands together for a few moments, bring your right hand to the root of your nose, between your two eyebrows.

- Using rapid movements with your right forefinger, tap your frontal chakra with the flat of your fingernail twelve times. This will create a feeling of pressure on the area.

- Slowly inhale as you try to feel this inhalation moving through the frontal chakra, like you're trying to fill an air pocket behind it. Repeat this inhalation a dozen times.

- Be cross-eyed internally without forcing it, but enough to create a feeling of pressure between your eyes. In the meantime, repeat the syllable "ta" loudly until you reach saturation (preferably no longer than one minute).

g) Purification of the Seventh Chakra

- Place both hands on your knees, palms up.

- Strive to perceive the presence of a white sun above your head. This sun will drop, one after another, seven droplets of gold onto your seventh chakra. Feel these seven droplets making contact on the top of your head.

- At your own pace, practice a few long breaths in and out.

- Visualize a kind of waterfall and the touch of the seven droplets on your head.

- At your own pace again, practice a few more long breaths in and out.

- Return to your perception of the droplets one last time.

- Take some time for inner silence, and then emit a long, deep buzzing sound from the back of your throat (or the traditional **Om** if you prefer).

h) Purification of the Eighth Chakra

Before beginning the eighth phase of this long practice, it will be helpful to refer to paragraph 5 of Chapter 3 of this book (p. 33).

- With both hands on your knees, palms up, observe a long silence while striving in the heart of this silence to perceive the sound of prana in you (a kind of hissing in the center of your head).

- Now try to perceive yourself about one meter (or 40 inches) "in the air" above your seventh chakra, almost like the location of a showerhead.

- When this mental image is created in your inner space and you have managed to "look down," drop a number of droplets of gold from the center of your consciousness to the top of your head under you (the top of the head that, of course, is yours).

- Finish this exercise with a long silence with both of your arms crossed at your chest, right over left.

Chapter III

The Disease Behind Its Mask

1) Autopsy the War

One of the first questions the priest-therapists of the Egypt of Akhenaten asked their patients was "Against whom or against what are you at war?" And in the same way, Christ frequently asked a question to those who sought healing from Him: "Tell me who your enemy is?"

These interrogations, which may surprise us today, give us an idea of the way the notion of illness was approached long ago.

Needless to say, when a sick person was presented with this question, his response was not guarded. It was not his body consulted at first but his soul, and this changed everything.

Within the Egyptian and Essenian fraternities, the approach was not to immediately analyze a symptom "through a magnifying glass." They sought rather to turn toward the world, very often mute, of causes.

It is then easy to understand that the disharmony that seizes a body is the result of an internal war that a being carries out, generally without knowing it, against a circumstance, others, or most often himself.

Why "generally"? In my opinion, it is the Master Jesus who best expressed the reason in a private interview with some of his disciples:

"Very often, I hear you blame the other person or the circumstances of your life when the illness takes possession of you. You cry out in incomprehension or about injustice, and you even lash out against our Heavenly Father. But what blindness, my friends! But what a lack of listening also to what you come across along your way! Is it not you who have generated, one after the other, each of the circumstances and encounters of your life? Is it not true that if you are standing in front of me now, it is because you have made choices and step in one direction rather than another? I am your circumstance for some form of health. Listen to me and believe me. We are always circumstances for each other. The pieces of a gigantic game that we attract to us or we push back. I mean that we are all, one next to the other, opportunities to grow or stagnate. We create the events by which we influence and reshape each other. Thus we make our balances and our imbalances. Our health opportunities as well as those of our diseases are the right fruits of the choices we make. The other, the one we accuse, is only the excuse behind which our blindness and our unconsciousness are hidden. The enemy, you see, is always something that we raise and feed steadily into ourselves. And we invent it in its totality because, in truth, it does not exist. Look at me and understand me. Of course, I am aware of opponents, but I have no enemy. Nothing in me or around me can be at war because I don't choose anything to apply force to or bring down. My health speaks of my peace. I weave my peace, and immediately I invent and reinvent myself, eternal and unassailable under the sun."

Such a speech, if we try to extrapolate its simplest meaning, speaks to us of only one thing: the feeling of unity that must preside over the physiological and psychological equilibrium of every person.

The perception of unity to be realized with the self and the world was really at the base of health as conceived in these traditions. Starting with this vision, a patient was therefore someone caught in a trap, that of duality and separation.

The resulting state of disruption and disharmony was seen as the creator of a certain number of scores or slashes in the consciousness, which extended quite naturally to the densest bodies.

In different terms, it was thought that the entrenchment of a state of conflict in a being almost inevitably became the origin of a future health disorder. This fits well with the modern notion of a "psychosomatic illness."

However, the traditional understanding of disease didn't stop there. There was also an exploration of a larger dimension of our universe—that of human thought and the energy reservoir it's made of.

Because of scientific measurement efforts, modern-day researchers believe the discovery of brain waves is a relatively recent development. These efforts, though, only placed a different word and some figures onto a reality already known to the ancient Egyptians. Those ancients and their successors knew very well that the simple act of thinking sets in motion impalpable and invisible forces that are not deprived of influence or real power over one's life. Also, the ancient Egyptians reckoned that each individual was surrounded by a wave of psychic life that followed him everywhere, something he was obviously projecting around him. But he was, above all, bathed in this wave, his overall health dependent on it.

2) Loft of Thoughts

This system of references also takes into account something else. The therapists started from the premise that the energy field of the human aura—since it is an energy field—is constantly interacting with our universe.

In fact, they were aware of the existence of an immense planetary aura on which the sum of the auras (the psychic activity of all of the Earth's inhabitants) interacts.

There existed for them "above" our visible world a universe, among others, comparable to a huge loft of thought. This colossal reservoir is composed of a large number of compartments. In each of them, all the seeds of a similar variety are lodged.

According to this concept, there exists, gathered on a specific vibrational plane, the energy mass of all your thoughts of anger. On another vibrational plane, all your thoughts of love are gathered. On another vibrational plane, all your thoughts of hatred exist. It goes on like this until the end of what humans are able to emit in beauty or not is reached.

Each of these vibrational planes corresponds to what we traditionally call an "egregore," or, in a modern way, a "morphogenic field." This acts as a receiver and at the same time a transmitter, the transmitter through which a human being resonates when he maintains in himself a certain state of thought and focus of consciousness.

In simpler terms, the ancients told us: "Talk anger, and you will be full of anger. Generate love, and you will be nourished with love. And if you feed the conflict, the conflict will come down in you, but if you sow sweetness, your path will end up being paved with unity."

3) A Force Called Coherence

One may argue nowadays that such a therapeutic approach was simplistic since everyone knows a disease may not spare people who practice good and healthy behaviors. Such a reality obviously was very well understood by the therapists of the past. Their understanding of the problem was based on *the principle of coherence.*

They felt that, whatever the level of consciousness and therefore behavior of a person, the way in which this person feels intimately unassailable, sure of himself and logical in his convictions, constitutes a kind of armor, more or less solid and resistant, prohibiting the creation of vibrational ruptures.

According to this theory, all it takes for a human to avoid disease is for him to perceive himself coherent and unbreakable within the aggressive manifestations of the illness. In a schematic way, we could say that the Egyptians and Essenians conceived of the fact that some people are able to simultaneously secrete their own poisons and antidotes.

Thus, when they approached a patient and questioned him about his "internal war," the therapists did not next "prescribe" a ritual intended to simply challenge the person in front of them. They listened intently to determine the level of coherence contained in the answers of the patient.

Indeed, we must recognize that many of us live constantly out of step with ourselves. There is, on one side, the way you see yourself, the way you dream of yourself, the way you want to be, and then on the other side, there is how you are able to embody the daily reality of the way you live. The degree of coherence or cohesion is, therefore, measured in the relationship between the inner world of a being and his or her external world.

What is also important to understand is that this degree of coherence—or inconsistency—is, more often than not, the responsibility of the individual person. We certainly cannot generalize, since the story of each of us is absolutely unique. But, at the least, gazing at one's positioning in life allows you to avoid slipping too easily into the heart of the great disease trying to legitimize all others—in other words, *victimization*.

4) The Disease-Entities

Let us now return to the notion of egregores and the "loft of thoughts," where some of the vibrational planes are filled with poisoned seeds. The Essenian fraternity developed a very particular approach.

It should be noted that this approach was not the result of some imaginary scaffolding aimed at satisfying a system of references, nor did it embody a set of hypotheses formulated by superstitious priests. It resulted from the direct experience of great mystics capable of projecting their consciousnesses far beyond our visible world.

These mystics managed to experience the detailed perception of the components of the etheric world and egregores that the human species have developed and maintained. The repeated study of these morphogenic fields, these egregores, and their levels (or vibrational planes) helped them understand that the mass of energy generated by a multitude of thoughts of the same type often ends up being inhabited and then controlled by embryonic life-forms generally derived from lower layers of the astral world or the ethereal world itself. According to this perception, this explains the birth of microorganisms called microbes or viruses.

Let's not forget that the conception of the microscopic world and the life that inhabits it does not date from the invention of microscopes. The atomic structure of matter had already been openly evoked in ancient Greece by Epicurus and, less well known, in India ten thousand years ago by a yogi named Kanada.

For the Essenian therapists, a disease with an infectious nature was therefore controlled by a kind of soul, although this is undoubtedly excessive. In reality, they spoke of the intelligence and relative autonomy of certain "psychic seeds."

According to the Essenians, the toxicity of a psychic seed (resulting in, for example, a virus) is linked to a form of intelligence creating these harmful entities that people have to deal with. Originating from this, specific rituals were created by the therapists, rituals we today view as magical.

But what is magic if not the perception and knowledge of the most intimate nature of our universe? And knowing how to master it by juggling with its wheels? This is not the science of the infinitesimally small but rather the infinitesimally subtle.

It is certainly not for me to direct research in this direction, which requires unusual qualities, but to provide clues for understanding for an enlargement of our field of concepts.

The Essenians were unmistakably distinguished from the Egyptians by the fact that they were very reluctant to use magical rituals. Their direction was one of the greatest possible starkness. In this sense, the emergence in their midst of an extraordinary therapist, Master Jesus, is obviously the pinnacle of what a human being can claim in such a field.

On this subject, I am regularly asked about the healing method put into practice by Master Jesus. Was it really that of the fraternity in which He had grown up?

Overall and in its main principles, yes. But the alignment and development of His subtle bodies were such that any technical element disappeared from His practice. In modern terms and schematizing somewhat, it seems today that it was enough for Him to send a message to His higher consciousness. He could then address a response to the subtle bodies of the being He was treating in order to trigger a process of healing. Most of the time, it was as easy as today making a phone call to the other side of the world.

With this in mind, it is important to remember that all of the elements of the techniques described in this book are first of all points of reference, a way to discipline oneself. They are of the same utility as the lines on the pages of a school notebook. They are also safeguards, or a hand extended to keep you from going too far in any direction. In no way do they represent the components of an absolute method, since all will be exceeded.

5) The Eighth Chakra

In a properly developed person, one can count seven levels of reality or consciousness. Each of them corresponds to a chakra and to the universe of that chakra. In Master Jesus, twelve levels of consciousness or realization were constantly manifesting, twelve levels in total communication with each other (which goes without saying).

The five levels of consciousness that distinguish a regular person from Him are those that still separate you from the revealed—or awakened—presence of your divine nature. When starting a flowering path such as that suggested, for example, in the practice of the therapies,[1] one should endeavor to understand that the five degrees of achievement in question are not states to be acquired. They are already present in seed form in each of us, waiting to be stimulated and then deployed one after the other over successive lives and times.

When an orchid branch starts to bloom, it is first the flowers buds closest to the base of the stem that open. The same goes for the "power plants" that are our chakras. From your reptilian, animal nature to your divine expansion, you will pass unmistakably through all stages of maturation. Thus, one's scale actually consists of twelve bars.

The major contribution of Pharaoh Akhenaten, then, even more brilliantly than that of Jesus, is the revelation to the West about the possibility of access to the eighth degree of the scale of a human being. This is the eighth chakra, the sun chakra of the Holy Spirit, that of the "supra mind" or higher self. It is in this direction that we move together. Whether you see it as a dove, a tongue of fire, a protective cobra, a crown, or a diamond matters little, because the Holy Spirit's essence in you will open each time you put your hand on a suffering being.

6) The Necessity Factor

We have spoken so far of disease as perceived by the ancients, as well as the principle of coherence, which opens more or less the door of the human organism. However, there is another factor involved in the field of health. It

---

1   *The Great Book of Essenian & Egyptian Therapies by Daniel Meurois & Marie Johanne Croteau.*

can be called the *necessity factor*. Indeed, the Egyptian and Essenian therapists considered that certain diseases are sometimes necessary in life for educational purposes. I use the word "educational" here in its most global sense. So I'm talking about an awakening, a purification, a reinitialization, a stimulation, an initiation, and a necessarily karmic rendezvous.

Indeed, in such a state of mind, the notion of a rendezvous is crucial. It is a temporary rendezvous, or one that leads to the destruction of the physical body but also an invitation to change your outlook on yourself and your life. It is a rendezvous through which you accept the teaching or against which you turn up with all your forces. But it is a rendezvous, finally, against which you can do nothing, since it was determined by the germs of the upper bars of your higher-self ladder—that is to say, by a wisdom that exceeds us all.

Understanding and then accepting what the law of karma represents is the key to all of this. Note that I place here understanding before acceptance because, very often, it is easier for one to understand the workings and the whys of a principle than to accept them when the effects are manifesting within. The integration, in one's flesh, of the necessity and the accuracy of a test requires a wisdom that only experience can bring gradually.

We must admit that a number of our health disorders— often the most significant—have no function other than that of encouraging us to "move." Shall you move for all that? That's the whole problem.

A door may be open. If you refuse to step through that doorway, you will stay where you are. The Divine, offering us opportunities for change, does not force us to live them. Thus, many diseases are, alas, simply experienced with suffering instead of being perceived as opportunities for growth.

The Egyptians knew that there are diseases that must be lived to the end. *No matter what a therapist is facing*, the Intelligence of Life plays fully its purifying and maturating role, even if physical death must be the outcome for a particular person.

For the Egyptians, most major health disorders were worth karmic rendezvous. It was therefore necessary to admit that they are endowed with a function and to respect it while not giving up when it comes to suffering.

It is important to understand that such an attitude is not fatalism. Indeed, the therapies were never interrupted; instead, they were supported by an increased moral presence and many soul-to-soul interviews with patients.

To illustrate this knowledge and respect for the laws that govern the equilibrium of an organism, I will quote Master Jesus again as an example. He, as we know, was constantly called to the bedsides of sick or dying people. But sometimes, he did not go to a place where he was asked to intervene. He simply answered that it was not the right time and that His Father would offer the person exactly what he needed. His spontaneous knowledge of individual karmas allowed Him to have such an attitude.

It is obvious that since humans cannot claim to have such an instantaneous ability to discern causes and necessities, we must nevertheless develop, beyond the constancy of our efforts, humility and wisdom in the face of the destiny of each one of us. "Destination" and "destiny" are words with the same origin, which suggests to us a route to follow. Let's try not to forget that.

7) The Intelligence of the Cell

Generally speaking, the compassionate dimension always allows the therapist to understand the meaning of a disease and its real significance. For that moment only, her art, still very flexible, is able to come into play as she finds issues leading to healing.

This may seem absurd today, but in their time, the Egyptians and Essenians claimed that the smallest part of an organ, a cell, needed to be talked about in a loving way. recognized the cell as an entity with intelligence and as permeable to love as to aggression, as well as capable of choosing unity or separation.

They also saw in every cell the meeting place, sometimes wounded and disharmonious, of five currents of force—two of a horizontal nature, associated with the positive and negative poles of the world of matter, and three of a vertical nature, generated by the triple Divine Essence.

With this in mind, the priest-therapists tried to be repairers, comforters, and simplifiers.

A disease, they said, is first the result of a conflict born of the complexity of the relationship with the living in the self.

Chapter IV

The Magic of the Oils

1) The Pharaoh and the Oils

"Let me tell you about the benefits of a specific marriage ... the one of the sun and the Earth. Indeed it is from this union that streams the great principle of the oil. Why am I talking about it? Because it is precisely the point of the ideal meeting between the subtle and the dense .... Both vertical and horizontal, it is the cobra that sneaks up everywhere ... it elevates everything while rising up. This is why I am asking you to look at one of the privileged receptacles of the Sacred."

These words were uttered by Pharaoh Akhenaten about 3,500 years ago. It is worth me sharing them today because they are certainly part of the rediscovery of some fundamental truths. Although he was not a therapist in the strictest sense of the term, Akhenaten fostered a vision of the universal order so "unitary" that he became an authority for all the priest-therapists of his time. It is indisputable that his conception of the sacred greatly influenced therapeutic practices, especially when it came to oils.

In breaking from the decadent clergy of Amon, the pharaoh also broke with a culture that had progressively desacralized the handling of certain substances, such as oils or odorous resins. The priests of Amon using oily substances in their religious rituals had indeed lost all sense. We could say today that they were painting religious statues with oil, but their gestures were in no way anointing anything. Their actions were meaningless, valueless.

The only real interest that was then taken in the use of oils revolved around massage and the exclusively physical enjoyment of the practice. In reality, Akhenaten's understanding was like that of a mystic constantly experimenting with higher states of consciousness. He did not strive to build an intellectually satisfying philosophical system for the sake of its own construction but rather communicated the direct fruit of his own discoveries. According to him, the oils represented the element by which the subtle and the sacred could sneak most easily into the heart of the dense.

He saw two reasons for this. First, there's the receptive character—how it's programmable (in today's language)—of an oil, and the second is its great ability to penetrate into a body.

For the intelligent and loving use of an oily material component, he reckoned that we could facilitate or amplify the descent of the solar Divine Principle into the heart of matter. This was, moreover, the basic reason for which, he asserted, the ancients anointed divine representations with oil.

With this anointing gesture, they were aware of inviting invisible principles to gradually inhabit the statues, thus modifying their vibrational rates, transforming them into "energy batteries" over the centuries. In this sense, a priest, just like a therapist today, occupied the height of what his role asked him to convey. He became a "pontiff" in the primary sense of the term—that is to say, a bridge builder.

It is obvious that an oil is only a working tool, and there is no power in it beyond its healing properties. A healing wave first passes, in absolute priority, through the heart and hands of a therapist.

The ancient signification of an oil as the union of the subtle and dense worlds is of great value for a therapist during a treatment. Oil is indeed a "plus," something that is useful and often pleasant to be able to count on.

2) The Vibrational Work of an Oil

My intention in this book is not to dwell on the subject of oils, since there are many specialized textbooks devoted to their properties and the curative function of their perfumes. In approaching this topic, it is my intention only to bring you my own testimony as to how I perceive the action of an oil at the level of the subtle bodies. I rely here on my perception of human auras. I've noticed that every time a therapeutic oil is deposited onto a part of the body, this immediately causes a kind of punctual bulge of the ethereal body. It is exactly as if the oil is called to an additional vital energy by a kind of magnetization phenomenon.

The bulge in question does not persist longer than two or three seconds. The ethereal "matter" then redistributes immediately, parallel to the skin. However, the skin's color will be modified according to the nature of the plants used in the creation of the oil. The color also depends on the amount of liquid placed on the targeted area of the body, and it may last for two or three hours, depending on the quality and degree of concentration of the plants used.

In the case of an essential oil, it is not uncommon to see the impact on the aura for twenty-four hours.

I would like to add that this aspect of the etheric counterpart of a zone is only the spectacular side of a more discreet phenomena, but it makes it possible to understand how an oil works.

Indeed, a much more "auric" perception of the anointed part of the body reveals that the energy wave of the oil sneaks into the peripheral nadis with an extraordinary speed sometimes, to the point of amazingly lightening them. The light, dispersed in the treated area, testifies to the precise information communicated to the prana, which receives it as a side effect and then communicates it into the blood and the cells.

We must not forget that the quality of the prana circulating in an organism, including its polarization (or the way it's loaded), greatly influences the quality of the blood. In fact, the blood and prana are closely related. The vibrational boundary that separates their respective worlds is permeable.

In some cases—and this is related to the quality of an oil and of course the work of a therapist—it is possible to see the energy wave of the oil going up through one nadi or more to the chakra director of the targeted organ. The chakra then reacts initially by opening and then redistributing, through the same nadis to the treated area, what I would call a big dose of "new prana," answering this call for help initiated by the particular oil.

When one has the ability to perceive this returning light wave, one notices that it is of a different color than that emitted by the oil in its movement toward the chakra. I personally perceive it as always being more of a pastel color and as coming to "extinguish" somewhat the vigor of the initial wave.

We can see that using a therapeutic oil is far from unimportant, even if this act is rarely enough on its own to obtain, nowadays, a total healing. I am saying "nowadays because our bodies are now adapted to rising amounts of chemical products of all kinds and consequently less receptive to the subtle help of oils and overall energy work.

The more ramparts are erected between the different vibrational levels of matter, the less these levels are able to interface with each other. The more we "fill a body," the more the body loses access to its roots from above.

When we are in possession of such information, we understand even more so that the use of an oil in a high concentration—the essence—must be done with caution. At high doses, essential oils dilate the nadis excessively, sometimes making them permeable and then capable of generating dispersions contrary to the desired effects. Similarly, an essential oil placed too generously and therefore illogically on a chakra may momentarily create an imbalance. You will see the chakra first dilate excessively, become irregular in its rotational movements, and then finally send jerky, disordered information to the network of nadis that it controls, possibly provoking sensations or unpleasant symptoms.

There is nothing dramatic that will happen, because the action of an oil is diluted in the space of a few hours, but such errors should not be repeated regularly to avoid setting in motion new troubles.

3) The Consecrated Oils

A few words now about consecrated oils. These oils are obviously not found in regular businesses, but they exist and some therapists use them.

After observing many times how a consecrated oil radiates, I cannot compare it to other oils. Its reach, and therefore its healing action, is considerably increased. This presupposes, of course, that the consecration of the oil was done consciously by a human being, a "priest in the soul"—in other words, someone playing the role of a bridge, as previously described.

True consecration is by no means a gesture connected with superstition or folklore. It is a call to a higher force, a force that is asked to descend.

All the truly consecrated oils I have been able to observe in use let out over them, once they are applied, a sort of bright cone of intense white light. The base of this cone is the size of the anointed area.

This luminous exhaust channel from the anointing oil, which has sometimes been perceptible to me up to fifty or sixty centimeters (twenty to twenty-four inches) away, makes me think, analogically, of a "coronal chakra" adapted to the oil. This coronal chakra is, of course, just an image, but it will help you get an idea of how the sacred aspect is implemented when using such a substance on the body.

As for the subtle bodies of a patient, these react differently when they receive a vibrational message from an oil that has been consecrated. There is mainly a large and harmonious expansion of the network of their nadis and a much longer persistence of the light wave conveyed through it.

The Egyptian and Essenian priest-therapists did not consider the use of non-consecrated oils. During some of their blessing rituals, they imprinted in individual oils the image of an archetype, a kind of example they could call on when visualizing, dreaming, or meditating.

It may be that they dedicated an oil especially for a patient and that their meditation and calling to this archetype were then directly focused on the patient's personality and symptoms. Behind each archetype, they saw the presence of a divine quality or function likely to counterbalance the disharmony installed in a suffering person.

Most of the archetypes that they let come to them were geometrically shaped. They affirmed, through the analysis of their own visions and also, for some, the practice of going out-of-body, that by diving into the heart of the infinitely subtle of any body, nothing other than living geometrical forms could be discovered.

According to them, these geometric forms organize themselves harmoniously or show signs of anarchy. The archetypes they called to go down into oils were supposed to act like conductors, able to resynchronize all of them.

All of this, of course, brings us directly to the words of Pythagoras, words that are carved on the front doors of some Greek temples: *"Let no one who cannot think geometrically enter here."*

In the Essenian community of Mount Krmel,[1] a kind of dictionary of oils existed. This highly specialized collection did not just list oils and describe their proper manufacturing from plants. It also indicated which archetypal geometrical form was immediately associated with this or that plant family and recommended the visualization for a selected archetype during the ritual of anointing an oil. The origin of this dictionary is Egyptian. The ones who developed this precious collection were the priest-therapists of the last years of Akhenaten's reign.

The Egyptian ideal was to revitalize an oil and its master plant by means of an archetypal geometrical form and then, in meditation and if necessary, to call for help from another archetype in relation to the imbalance of the sick person.

Some nowadays wrongly claim that the Essenian therapists feared oils and did not practice anointing. This claim comes from a warning of some Essenians, in particular in Qumran in what is now Israel, in reaction against those called the "magicians of the desert," who did not hesitate to load dark energy into oily substances to satisfy their "customers."

Be that as it may, the complete and detailed science of the Egyptian association of the archetypes of plants and oils no longer seems accessible today, although some researchers are working to restore it. The consecration of oils, though, remains more within our reach.

By mentioning in this chapter the existence of oils already consecrated and whose quality is remarkable, this does not mean that it is necessary to rush to research them and only use them. Indeed, by definition, their production and distribution are extremely limited.

On the other hand, according to the Egyptian-Essenian healing approach, every human being whose heart is pure and who perceives him- or herself without lies or artifice as a

---

1   *See Chapter IV, The Way of the Essenes: Christ's Hidden Life Remembered.*

therapist is perfectly capable of achieving a consecration. At this level, each person is acquainted with their own sincerity, lucidity, and especially perception and willpower in pursuit of unconditional love and service to others.

The efficiency of a consecration depends on the quality of the bridge. A ritual is by no means a recipe. Above all, it is the way by which a therapist precisely directs a wave of love.

4) Consecration of the Oils

To do this, the Egyptians and Essenians used a "mudra." A Sanskrit word, these are body positions that call and concentrate divine, psychic, or even simply ethereal energies. In more modern and schematic terms, mudras generate energy circuits aimed at developing and polarizing different levels of the body with specific forces. Some are complex and result from sustained yogic practice, while others are within everyone's reach, if carried out consciously.

The Mudra of the Consecration, as used formerly, is a very simple action by itself. It comes down to arching the index finger by raising its end with the help of the middle finger, as indicated in the drawing below.

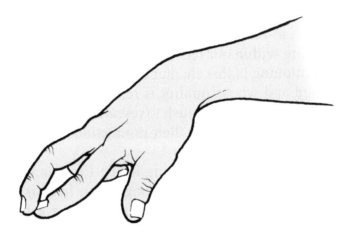

With the help of this position of the fingers, the priests of Akhenaten drew ankhs[2] in the air and in the direction of the body or part of the body to be sacralized. They usually drew three ankhs and then kept the mudra fixed toward what they were blessing. This was the chosen moment during which, with closed eyes, they visualized the archetype that had previously been revealed to them.

It is possible to consecrate an oil in the most general sense—that is, without dedicating it to a precise healing function or to a sick person in particular. In this case, the assistance of an archetype is not used, unless one comes spontaneously to impose itself behind your closed eyelids. You will make this be a moment of intimate prayer or emptiness, according to your heart's disposition.

I want to emphasize that, although this mudra requires a little physical exercise with your fingertips, it is essential to learn how to achieve it without tensing. The less muscular tension there is, the more the wave of consecration escaping from the index and middle fingers will be fluid and powerful.

Some may also perceive the wave in the form of a ray that is white, green, or blue. This ray will "caress" the oil to about twenty centimeters (about eight inches) in front to energize and sacralize it.

5) The Olfactory Dimension of Oils

The olfactory dimension was not neglected by the ancients. The Egyptian therapists, however, used it more than their Essenian inheritors, who again showed themselves to always be in search of a greater plainness. According to Akhenaten's therapists, the creation of an olfactory ambiance was important for any healing treatment in a consecrated room.

---

2   *The ankh (the "cross of life" or "crux ansata") is an ancient Egyptian hieroglyphic cross symbol with a loop for its top arm. Among the Coptic Egyptians, it was defined by a circular loop.*

We know how it is often unpleasant today, or very painful, to walk through the corridors of hospitals. The smell of food is mixed with that of disinfectants, and the air circulating is saturated with heavy, artificial fragrances. The generally incoherent search for a certain sanitization leads to the almost systematic retraction of the auras of all those living in such a context.

The retraction of an aura is always an automatic protection measure initiated by the subtle organism. It reflects the fact that a body is "on guard," on the defensive, which is basically the opposite of the attitude needed for a healing solution.

In a pictorial way, I would say that the auric egg protects itself by "solidifying" in the presence of certain odors.

This is not about something subjective or secondary. There are entities that open and others that close an organism to a flow of healing. The Egyptians spoke willingly of the light of a perfume or an odor.

For them, it was a little of the soul of the "deva,"[3] or the director, of the used plant absorbed by the nostrils. In their eyes, this type of communion with an odor pointed to the origin of the expansion or retraction of the aura.

The olfactory atmosphere of their therapy rooms was perceived as essential, constituting the first stage at which the subtle bodies of a sick person become more open.

It goes without saying that each of us is different in perceiving smells, and some have allergies to certain types of perfume. The reasons for this are so numerous that it is impossible to describe them all here.

Generally speaking, even though you may be used to a specific incense in your therapy space before a treatment, it is important and respectful to ask the person who has come to be healed if what she is breathing suits her.

---

3   *See p. 31, The Portal of the Elves by Marie Johanne Croteau-Meurois.*

The same rule applies to oils. The ancient therapists did not perform anointings with scents that fundamentally displeased their patients. For them, it was not just a question of "olfactory comfort." They knew that doors would be closed to those they cared for if what they breathed in was not pleasant to them.

The chakra most affected by odors and perfumes is undoubtedly the root chakra. Our sense of smell can be described as being the most animal-like of all. It is logical, then, that it is associated with the first of our subtle centers, which is, by nature, connected in a privileged way to the Earth Element, our basic chakra.

Animals feel before seeing. They perceive very precisely the aura of a being through the fragrant emanations of it.

The radiating of the root chakra is not easy to visualize because of its location in the most intimate part of the human body. It is certain, however, that a well-suited oil, which the patient will appreciate, will greatly contribute to dilating it. The "grounding" of the organism will thus be facilitated, a sizable step for a return to health.

There is the impression that a perfume only concerns the respiratory sphere of one's being and that it influences it by involving the laryngeal chakra.

This, however, represents only an apparent and partial aspect of things. The chakra of the throat, the fifth, is just a door. It is the major transit route used by a perfume and its information to penetrate quickly into a body. But, in fact, it is the whole body, with its multiple layers, that absorbs the odorant information to convey it a second time to the base chakra.

When the first chakra has absorbed the essence of the perfume and expanded by connecting more to the Earth Element, it will be able to redistribute the information received to the entire body by way of the appropriate nadis.[4]

---

4   See pgs. 28–30, *The Great Book of Essenian & Egyptian Therapies* by *Daniel Meurois & Marie Johanne Croteau.*

Chapter V

A Multidimensional Therapy

1) The Physical Dimension

In the field of the subtle energy therapies introduced in this book, especially when it comes to their sacred aspect, it is not uncommon to note that a certain duality is still well established.

I am referring to the famous—and fake—body-spirit opposition. In other words, this is the focus on the immaterial origin of a health disorder to the point that the body is not even considered, barely touched with an anointing oil. Such a therapeutic approach brings a full disembodied aspect to a healing session.

Certainly, this approach can make sense and ensure great results. I myself can confirm this as a witness. However, this direction is not an option with regard to the work methods of the Egyptians and Essenians. According to those therapists, a human being is only complex in appearance. A human was not definitively divided because matter and spirit were not seen as antagonists.

The three principles—body, soul, and spirit—overlapped, communicated, and definitely did not contradict one another.

As a human being was, obviously, considered a higher and spiritual blueprint, his body was respected as a lengthening of the subtle bodies and a tool for growth.

Could there be great sculptors without the proper hammers or chisels? Could there be great painters without color palettes or brushes? The most prodigious of creators generates nothing without the extension of her consciousness through something more dense, which she accomplishes herself.

So the ancient therapists were not afraid of the physical human reality. Actually, they learned to closely examine the energy of an organism.[1]

They knew to enter into direct contact with it. They did not ignore the fact that most sick people are sensitive and even very receptive to the physical touch of hands on their bodies.

Taboos relating to the body were much less relevant than one imagines, and infinitely less numerous than those that developed later in the Judeo-Christian civilization. The human body was by no means seen as scandalous, and the therapeutic touching approach was, in principle, not viewed as indecent.

This does not mean, however, that what are now called "blockages" or "inhibitions" were then unknown. In fact, any society is capable of inventing its own taboos, prohibitions, and internal conventions, which necessarily cause psychocorporal imbalances.

All of this is to say that the therapists of which I make myself the spokesperson today were aware of the importance of tactile, direct contact between one who cares and his patient. They asserted that the quality of heat and radiance of the palm of a hand resting on a body spoke a language as determinative as that of a loving gaze offered at a "soul-to-soul" distance.

In reality, they were aware of two things. First of all, some sick people need to be touched physically. Secondly, it is up to the therapist, and generally an individual, to overcome the limitations erected between the multiple levels of the mindset

---

1   See p. 52, *The Great Book of Essenian & Egyptian Therapies* by Daniel Meurois & Marie Johanne Croteau.

conditioning experienced in life. According to this approach, the body is able to express what is in the soul and spirit in the body's language. This vision is, consequently, one of unity and therefore unitary.

How could the different degrees of the same original reality escape or even fight each other? This was one of the first topics of reflection submitted to students with regard to the art of healing. But let's go back to the issue of touch as a possible vehicle for a wave of healing. In discussing the basic findings of the Egyptian therapists, I mentioned the overwhelming need of some patients to be touched physically. This statement is not too strong, I believe.

Indeed, in all cultures (and for sometimes opposing reasons), many people have become gradually "separated" from their own bodies. This has gone on since the beginning of time. These people do not really inhabit their bodies because of a lack of external stimulation. I am not talking here of romantic stimulation. This is another area, one simply of loving stimulation, of a spontaneous contribution of love capable of enlivening the cells of the body.

Any attentive therapist knows how much her hand just placed on a forehead, a rib cage, a belly, or even a wrist can automatically trigger a flood of liberating tears. Why? Because the body happens to forget that it exists, that it is to be respected, loved, and, finally, that the most beautiful dimensions of the being also need to express themselves through the physical body.

Your spirit, your soul, and your body make up a wholeness, but one of them is repressed or forgotten. Suffering thus takes place, with many symptoms.

Part of the art of healing, therefore, consists of knowing which needs direct contact with a caring hand(s) more than the others.

In a general way, and according to my own memories and observations, the ancient therapists used physical touch almost systematically. On the one hand, the use of oils pushed them, while on the other hand, they noticed that certain precise points or areas of the body act as levers, releasing important tensions. They understood that certain assemblages of cells act like locks, behind which painful memories are incarcerated, reflexes of the injured soul.

How did they find these areas of injury? By being attentive to the quality of a patient's skin and its heat, from one area to another.

Here are some of their basic observations. It goes without saying that these are only indicative or reflective paths, not absolute truths.

a) The Temperature of the Body

A cold area on the surface of the body was considered akin to an obvious lack of vital breath. A therapist would therefore inquire about the health of a patient's gut, as well as the major nadis running through the major organs in the belly. This questioning could, of course, lead one to consider the activity of the driving chakra of the area identified. It was also noted that there is a need to differentiate between a dry and wet cold. This distinction requires a little practice and especially attention from the therapist.

A dry cold usually indicates a lack of love or affection from the consciousness to the indicated area. An emotional shock can also provoke it.

A wet cold signifies, for its part, a loss of energy of a "mechanical" origin. It is mainly noticed as a result of punches, injuries, or surgeries. Consequently, some nadis may be damaged, severed, or entangled.

It may also be necessary to notice an excess of heat at a precise point on the skin. In any case, this perception will connote a massive influx of prana. If the area has not been physically stimulated by a muscular exercise, it is likely that, for some reason to be determined, we are dealing with the congestion of an important nadi.

At the junction point of some nadis, sorts of "energy switches" shut down. The causes can be very diverse: bad food, a microbial infection, or even simply an emotional shock. This is because any point of the body can have a symbolic value or refer to a memory for each individual.

In this labyrinth to be disentangled, it is obviously essential to seek out the simplest possible causes before digging ourselves deeper in the background of the consciousness.

b) The Quality of the Skin

It is easy to understand that soft, supple skin represents globally harmonious or simply coherent functioning.

It is thus important to identify possible points of tension, stiffness, or dryness. These always speak to an accumulation of etheric waste.

Such wastes secreted by the subtle organism can, at first, be eliminated by small, vigorous, circular massages practiced in a counterclockwise direction. Of course, it will be necessary to look at the root cause of the waste accumulation.

Before making a psychological diagnosis, one must first consider the possibility of much simpler causes, such as injury or bad positioning of the body related, for example, to a regular activity. It is not uncommon to search very far for what is within reach of immediate comprehension—in other words, to ignore one's own common sense.

It should be noted that tension and dryness on the skin of a woman often indicates a lack of emotional support or self-esteem and frequently reveals hormonal issues.

Let us not forget that each of the remarks made here about the state of skin is only valid if the condition persists or repeats itself over time. Many are episodic and therefore insignificant.

To return to simplicity and common sense, I will tell you here another story related to the life of the great Egyptian therapist Sinuhe,[2] renowned for performing miracles through the laying on of his hands.

He was once called to one of the women belonging to the aristocracy of the city of Akhetaton. The lady in question had split open her forearm after sliding down a stone staircase. Proud of her beauty, she was panicked. She believed that if Sinuhe did not intervene with his so-called miraculous abilities, she would forever have an unsightly scar on her arm.

At her bedside, he looked at the wound for a few moments and then went away. He came back with a sort of plaster made of crushed herbs and milk. Without saying anything, he applied the bandage around her forearm. "Is that all?" asked the young woman, a little peeved. Her name was Ner-Taru. "That's all," Sinuhe answered her. "Let us give each world what belongs to it. Sometimes, the flesh only demands the language of the flesh."

2) The Psychological Dimension

Most dysfunctions of the body are complaints of the soul.

This was the basic assumption of the ancient therapists, a truth that we are rediscovering today. With this awareness, one should not think of approaching a treatment without proper contact with the client. Every suffering person who enters in a therapeutic place hoping to be healed wants to be listened to, heard, and understood above all.

According to the ancient conception, a client must feel an aura open in front of him and embrace it in its totality. This aura is a sanctuary and obviously the therapist's. A sign on the door will not create this aura. It is cultivated in the crucible of compassion, a compassion that starts with respect.

Anyone who visits a therapist is in a state of fragility. The Egyptian priests taught their students to never contradict a suffering person. Instead, you listen to her patiently, even

---

2   *La Demeure du Rayonnant (Home of the Radiant Sun) by Daniel Meurois.*

if what she says is incoherent or seems to be the fruit of her imagination.

It is too common nowadays for a doctor to mock a patient or dismiss his statements with a simple brush of the hand while stating that what he's suffering from "does not exist," that it's "psychological." Such an attitude is not only dismissive but also indicative of a basic ignorance of human beings.

A psychological disorder is not "nothing." It can lead to real suffering that, though difficult to quantify, needs to be considered. A pain of the soul, even if it is claimed that it is not based on anything, is sometimes very quickly enough to unbalance an organ or a whole system.

Taking great care to not contradict a suffering person does not mean the therapist believes her story. It is simply about showing that she is being taken seriously and accepted, despite all the possibly incoherent "pieces" she may share. This establishes the foundation for mutual trust essential for a real dialogue. When there are mental constructions to be unraveled, these will then be approached gradually and in a simple way.

But how does one learn compassion? Here is some Essenian wisdom: *"Listening and sharing from the heart are like fruits that grow only on a patiently pruned tree for many seasons and for many years.*

If you see the flowers in the spring, do not expect to reap the benefits in the following fall. It takes many lives to fully bear a name and offer it to the world."

This truth, based on observation, enables us to understand why the art of the therapy is taught and learned only to a certain extent, and where the art of healing begins. From the moment when a simple and spontaneous love springs up in a therapist and she becomes able to transmit it, she stops fighting a disease and begins to feed the health—and life—of a patient.

3) The Emotional Dimension

Whatever is done, the emotional dimension exists as soon as a relationship of trust is established at the core of a treatment. Faced with a real health disorder—physical and psychological—Egyptians and Essenians felt their role was to take the hand of the man or woman in pain to bring them out of shifting sands to firm ground.

In doing so, they knew about the existence of a major trap inherent to the role of helper.

By pointing out a path of transformation, by becoming the initiator of metamorphosis, an ancient therapist had already understood the phenomenon of what we now call "transfer." This is sometimes described as an excessive focus of the client's thoughts toward the human personality of the therapist and a possible transfer of affection, especially when therapist and patient are of opposite sexes, which is easily understandable. Whether we speak of ancient or modern times, every human being functions identically. It is the same great psychological and emotional resources that make him react. It was not uncommon in the Temple of the Therapies in the city of Akhetaton for priest-therapists to test the emotional balance of their students. They would entrust the students with certain patients and observe the evolution of treatments among them.

The students readily demonstrated the rise of the transfer phenomenon.

In some cases, some apprentice-therapists were trapped in challenging circumstances. For example, the emotional connection with a particular client had become an obstacle to treatment. This happened for two reasons. First, the therapist no longer had sufficient distance from the person they were treating, and secondly, the patient, more or less consciously, understood that the cessation of his or her suffering would mean the loss of the connection with the therapist.

It should be recognized that, for some patients, there is a comfort within a disorder. The health problem becomes the person's universe. They use it and find satisfaction in it, if only by means of care and a consoling emotional presence.

The priest-therapists felt that such a situation is never totally avoidable because it's based on the foundations of human nature. When there is a holistic approach to treatment— body, soul, and spirit—and the integration of a patient's health history, fears, doubts, physical ailments, and any questions, the patient is never viewed as just a disease or symptom but rather as a person. He is a man or she is a woman to heal, a being to be considered and loved for the divine part dwelling within him or her. The teaching that was then provided by the priest-therapists included long hours of discussion devoted to shining light on the stalemates that could occur between therapists and patients.

Before the development of modern psychology, Egyptian teachers noticed that a therapist who offers a treatment almost automatically takes on a paternal dimension in the subconsciousness of the patient. This dimension forms a force as it generates at the same time a fragility. This force-fragility duo is closely interrelated in any human relationship, in the center of which the presence of each person's heart is tangible.

As soon as one enters into a deep relationship of trust and begins to love, whether it's true love, tenderness, or friendship, one connects to the reinvigorating source while being totally opened to a certain vulnerability.

Reading the Akashic records enabled me to understand that 2,000 years ago, Master Jesus had to deal with the phenomenon of transfer several times. As a result of some of His miracles, He found Himself confronted with emotional overflowing on the part of some women. He tried to get away with words and smiles of appeasement, but nothing helped.

We cannot ask the sun to look like the moon. We just need to be aware of what it is and move forward in life with, again, the maximum of common sense.

To return to the paternal dimension of the therapist, the Egyptian priests confirmed the possibility of a merger with the maternal dimension for a therapist who deploys compassion in their work. The father-mother image is then imposed on both the patient and his or her therapist. This clearly shows that the therapist enters a state of wholeness, even mastery.

At this stage of perception and connection, the phenomenon of affective attachment presents less risk in terms of human relationships because, by increasing his healing skills, the therapist becomes asexual. Then, too, in the course of the healing that he embodies, the therapist is increasingly perceived as a teacher and guide by the patient. In the same way, a therapist does not have to work against a possible attitude of rejection or loss of confidence on the part of the patient being treated. This person is not "his" patient. The therapist is in a kind of relay in the life of the sick person. She has the mission of helping the patient to a certain point, after which she must hand off her efforts.

Of extreme importance is taking the "temperature" of the soul of the suffering person after each treatment.

The ancient therapists felt it was important to feel regularly where a patient is, beyond the idea of the pattern of treatments that was subsequently seen. They learned to constantly question their "ideal protocol" based on the reactions of the sick people they were helping. This was so a patient would never feel locked into a mandatory process and trapped.

There is no real healing, nor an advance toward any liberation whatsoever, without total freedom of the soul.

4) The Spiritual Dimension

The spiritual dimension is the direct, and I would say indispensable, extension to all that has just been described in this book.

A properly provided series of healing sessions will open the soul of a patient to another perception of herself and life itself.

In this sense, beyond the concrete aspect of treatments, a therapist worthy of the name draws new doors in the consciousness of those he receives, and he guides them without forcing any passages. To guide is to precede, to unravel a path in order to clear a horizon, not to push the person in front of you because you think you know where he or she should go.

This does not exclude firmness, however, because softness without firmness easily becomes sluggishness and laziness. A guide also shows the pitfalls.

The denunciation of these difficulties, which does not always suit the person to whom it is addressed, must be clearly pronounced and updated regularly. If this were not the case, it would quickly lead to a kind of "purring" of the consciousness within a "marshmallow-colored" treatment on a boring path.

A health disorder is always an occasion, even an explicit proposal, for a metamorphosis. It suggests a change in the soul and the updating of its operating mode. All the skills of the therapist are utilized in her understanding the nature of this change and then facilitating the process, with the help of her own radiance and the rightness of the words that she lets come to her.

All this has certainly become commonplace in personal development circles, but in recalling the basics in a few words here, my goal is primarily to point out the responsibility of the therapist in such a process. The role of the therapist is not necessarily that of a guide, defined as a "soul midwife." In learning this function—learning that never stops—it is up to each therapist to know how to recognize and admit his or her own limits.

It is a greatness to admit incompetence or a lack of perception or preparation in this or another field. It is a greatness too to know when to refer someone to another therapist. And it is a dangerous pettiness to pretend to possess a mastery that one has not yet developed.

In this regard, the priest-therapists of ancient Egypt willingly subjected their students to tests that could be called unfair but at least had the merit of exposing abuses of power. The abuse of power is unquestionably a deadlock into which any therapist can sink when he reaches a certain stage of his practice. This attitude can lead him to take himself too seriously, resulting in a mental sickness called sufficiency.

This is one of the classic traps Egyptian students faced when instructors suspected excessive tendencies taking over. They would hire a comedian and ask him to simulate certain well-defined symptoms. Over a number of weeks, he was asked to note the overall behavior of particular apprentice-therapists toward him. Any deviance or abuse of power on a therapist's part was consequently quite easily exposed.

Thus, one did not become a full priest-therapist until after a long period of study and various probations highlighting not only technical knowledge but also, above all, the qualities of harmony, uprightness, and kindness. In sum, the goal was a realization of being human in the fullest sense of the word.

A student was greatly tested and challenged both in his body and his soul during all the years of training. This was normal, since the function to which he was destined was sacred. Can we say the same today?

By helping a person overcome their mental creases, dissolve their emotional pockets, and clean their cell memories, they become necessarily invited to completely renew their perception of who they are and their relationship to the world. The therapist thus becomes the initiator and stimulator of a new spiritual dawn, even if this expression scares a few.

That is why, at a certain point in the healing process, it is not uncommon for a patient to experience unusual phenomena, such as visions while in a waking state, sensations of burning localized on a chakra or chakras, jolts of energy running down the back to the tailbone followed by headaches, or overwhelming dreams. These phenomena and others not mentioned here are classic and logical. Nevertheless, it is essential that the therapist know how to help her patient navigate such a disconcerting jungle.

"Dedramatizing" is certainly the key word to never lose sight of when such situations arise. These experiences are, fortunately, fleeting. Faced with them, and for the purpose of appeasement, the therapist must identify through ethereal palpation[3] and aura reading (if possible) the area(s) of the patient's body that's still comparable to a switch in the "off" (or closed) position.

Increasingly, I have noticed the beginnings of awakening the Kundalini force among those who use subtle-energy treatments. The manifestations that this generates are to be taken with the greatest seriousness because the power of the triple fire housed at the base of the spine can unleash in the human body an energy comparable to an atomic bomb. In the beginning of this process, the person will have the painful impression that he is going toward his own dissolution, all in the midst of the most varied and indefinable physical pains.

Obviously, one must not mess around with the Kundalini awakening. It is not a matter, then, of going against its development but rather controlling it through the work of liberation and openness. This work will be performed by the therapist at the levels of the seventh and fourth chakras simultaneously.

In general, it is important to understand that the first chakra should never be powerfully worked on without being certain that the dorsal axis is properly disengaged and that the seventh chakra is sufficiently deployed to absorb the shock caused by a rise in Kundalini energy.

The phenomenon is easy to understand by thinking of a fireplace. To be able to make fire in a fireplace, it is necessary first that the hatch of the fireplace be opened. (This is akin to

---

3   See pgs. 61–63, *The Great Book of Essenian & Egyptian Therapies* by
    Daniel Meurois & Marie Johanne Croteau.

63

ensuring a healthy base in the patient to be treated.) Secondly, the conduit of this fireplace must be swept. (The energy axis of the patient's spine is without a zone of retention, or very clean.) And third, nothing should come close to the top of the fireplace at the level of the roof, like a bird's nest for example. (In other words, the patient has the real ability to achieve higher awareness with real aspirations.)

One can easily understand that when all of these conditions are not met, smoke will flow back to the heart of the house and invade it.

In the worst-case scenario, this will also cause a fire (or the burning of the patient's conduit and, perhaps, the whole "house").

When one is obviously faced with the profound energy transformation of a human being, wisdom recommends doing nothing to speed up the pace. Be happy to be the regulator and a patient therapist. You must avoid the explosion or energy implosion of a patient's body. The required transformation will take place on its own, passing from one organ to another throughout the body, often painfully but in a safe way because this is natural.

The result of all this will be a faster circulation of prana in the whole body and, hence, an increase of its vibrational rate, as well as a more perfect alignment with the higher consciousness from which it comes, a guarantee of a real inner awakening.

Part Two

Chapter VI

The Foundations of the Therapies

1) An Aura Reading?

Let us continue to refer to the wisdom of those who preceded us in ancient times. Grasping this wisdom, as it has been said many times, regularly involved the practice of reading the human aura as a tool for diagnosis and prevention.

Does this mean that all ancient therapists mastered the art of viewing the subtle bodies? Certainly not. Even if the emissions of radiances generated by human beings back then were clearly more perceptible than nowadays (due to less psychic pollution of the planet), many therapists were unable to access such knowledge, at least beyond a certain level of perception.

In addition, I want to point out that those who navigated with ease the practice of reading the bodies did not, however, systematically engage in aura reading as soon as sick people presented themselves.

The reason for this is very simple. It can be summed up in two points. The first involves the personality of the patient.

The psychological approach must be taken into consideration to try to guess her level of "mentalization" not only of her own problems but also of the impact of the therapist's words on her.

It goes without saying that a very cerebral person will react intellectually to an aura reading. Instead of letting the essence of his being assimilate what is revealed to him, he will dissect, sometimes for weeks, the "state of the premises" that the therapist has discovered. In such a case, nothing will be settled because the patient will tend to focus excessively on what has been revealed to him rather than allowing his soul and his cells to calmly digest the revealed information, as it should be.

The Essenians, with all their delicacy, certainly were more aware of this aspect of things. Faced with a suffering person's very mentally focused behavior, they practiced aura reading only to a certain point in advancement of a treatment, if at all. They thus intended not to distort the healing process by avoiding the slightest possibility of crystallization of a patient's psyche on the conditions of his difficulties.

In light of all this, it is easy to understand that the light and liberation usually accessible from a detailed reading of the aura only pays off for someone capable of, at a minimum, letting go, relaxing, and listening to their inner self.

The integration of an aura reading into a process of healing therefore requires the patient to let go, open up to all eventualities, and, finally, trust.

The second reason that an aura reading was not necessarily practiced from the outset with a patient is that when a therapist wishes to obtain a truly accurate map of the subtle bodies and their interactions, it is preferable to proceed with a preliminary cleaning. When an aura reading is being considered, a first encounter with a patient should ideally conclude with a treatment aimed at liberating the subtle organism from as much of its pollution (its "etheric waste") as possible.

At the second meeting, a more detailed reading of the energy organism can be undertaken.

To return to the Essenians, it is certain that they did not abstain at any given moment in a series of treatments and were able to review each situation by means of a new aura reading. As with the Egyptians, their ultimate goal was always to leave the door completely open for the patient so that she, ideally, could manage to make her own diagnosis. They sought to bring her little by little to an awareness of her own internal difficulties. In a general way, it was not a matter of announcing to someone, "I see that you are that!" Instead, it was important to take time when sharing what was perceived, and this was always done with kindness and consideration. Reading an aura was handled like rational research.

These specifics do not go against the principles of an aura reading. On the contrary, this encourages practicing a reading in a fairer way because of the more refined approach. This is a warning about the tendency that some might have to rely on their own perceptions of patients as absolute truths. Let us remember that the impact of a diagnosis, in whatever form it may be, may be considerable. A person who sees herself stuck with a label of this or that disorder in a categorical way can end up more mired in her original problem.

For ancient therapists, a reading of the subtle bodies was only a method of approach, a suggestion, a basis of reflection from which one worked with a patient to deepen a search or confirm or refute a situation.

Today, the basic rule remains the same. Even if you are certain, it is not up to you to impose this certainty. You would be a potential jailer instead of an instrument of liberation.

2) The Role of Oil

When taking into account all that has been said before about the impact of oils,[1] it is logical then to use them only after an aura reading. This is simply because the vibration

---

1   See Chapter Four, "The Magic of the Oils."

of an oil is, most of the time, very powerful, and it could disturb a reading. The presence of an oil can interfere with one's perception of the subtle bodies.

The Egyptians, well versed in their art, sometimes anointed the forehead of a patient with a balm composed of three resins, including frankincense (or olibanum). This anointing was practiced on someone whose aura did not "open" to a reading and remained compressed on itself, like a closed hand fan, by reflex of protection, whether conscious or not.[2]

The composition of such a balm is probably lost today, but there is an essential oil whose action is comparable when it is placed, sparingly, on the frontal chakra. It is the essential oil of hemlock (*Tsuga canadensis*), a tree considered to be the largest evergreen conifer in North America.

Its relaxing power can greatly help the deployment of contracted auras. This oil is, however, not a systematic remedy to the problem mentioned here. Many auras resist despite the usage of this oil, reminding us that there is no need to insist on it.

3) Saliva

Saliva was used regularly, both by the Egyptians and Essenians, at the beginning of each session. The therapist melted a small quantity of his saliva with a little soil taken by the sick person from where he lived.

This mixture was gently placed in an anointing at the top of the forehead, at the median root of the hair, and also at the point of the body that was suffering, if it could be clearly located. In this way, it was used in bridging to create an impact, an opening.

The reason is simple. Saliva holds an extraordinary concentration of prana. Much of the vital energy of a being

---

2   *See p. 67, Les Maladies Karmiques (The Karmic Diseases) by Daniel Meurois.*

is concentrated in his or her saliva. This is one of the reasons why lovers feel the need to kiss each other. The mixture of their fundamental energies, if only at this level, strengthens their beings by establishing a point between the subtle and the dense.

Mixed with a little soil, saliva serves as an amplifier of the energy of the Earth Element. It increases the harmony in the existing vibration between the subtle bodies and the sick person.

The mixture created by saliva and soil likely caused quite surprising effects. In a general way, it was placed on the area concerned in long and slow movements in the form of a lemniscate, or infinity symbol (∞). Gesturing in the shape of a lemniscate generates an engine, a multiplication. The infinity symbol is an accelerator that acts directly on the circulation rhythm of the prana by condensing it. In the basic initiatory teaching of the priests, it was said that the lemniscate could be thought of as a representation of the cosmic engine specific to the grand universe. It is made by two movements: one of gathering and another of dispersion or dissolution. An inhale and then an exhale. It represents, at its symbolic level, a way of translating the famous alchemical principle "solve et coagula," which means dissolve and coagulate.

The use of saliva is, of course, much more tricky today, especially in Western society. For reasons of hygiene, it is indeed immediately considered suspect, and therefore, it cannot be used at the outset of a treatment.

Does this mean that it must be totally abandoned? That would be a real shame, because its virtues are indisputable.

The solution is asking for the patient's consent and taking the time to explain the reasoning behind this method. It goes without saying that with a little basic training in psychology, a therapist will know very quickly to whom he can or cannot offer such a contribution within a treatment. The golden rule is always to not cause discomfort or awkwardness. Delicate procedures should be very freely consented to in a global process of trust.

4) Which Side of the Body?

And why not on the three sides of the body? This is indeed what was advocated by those who serve as a reference in this book. They treated the back, the front, and also the profile.

When the physical condition of a patient allowed her to easily lay on her stomach, the back was always the starting point. In a human being, the majority of difficulties, among other things, will be reflected by back tightness in multiple areas. For the ancient Egyptians, it was therefore inconceivable to start a treatment without having first undertaken a dissolution, or at least a reduction, of such tensions.

Moreover, the dorsal axis—the spine—constitutes the true "tree of life" of a human being. The state of the chakras is easily perceptible there and often more neutral than on the front of the body. On this subject, I strongly recommend analyzing the color of the skin in the region of each chakra, especially in the coccygeal and cardiac regions. It is not uncommon, especially nowadays, for people experiencing huge and numerous changes to have significant redness in these areas.

In extreme cases, an area of redness may reproduce the archetypal pattern of a chakra (a triangular figure or a specific star, for example).

This is always a sign of the overactivation of the center on which the pattern appears. It must be taken into consideration because it indicates a real "overheating" of the subtle organism and can be at the source of important disorders or at least very unpleasant ones, like intense burning sensations, nausea, fever, vertigo, and headaches. Most of the time, such cutaneous manifestations are due to too much stimulation of the chakras involved. Stimulations of an emotional order are sometimes caused by excessive, uncontrolled, and even inappropriate practices of meditation, visualization, or concentration. Once again, a phenomenon of this type, only temporary, will not have any significant characteristics. If it persists, it is something else.

It happens, of course, that such red areas, sometimes accompanied by small, even redder dots, appear from time to time on the front of the body, including on the fourth, fifth, and sixth chakras. They should not be given more consideration because they are "in the front" and therefore more eye-catching. In general, the Essenians and Egyptians noticed that the discoloration of skin on a chakra was more episodic and emotionally rooted when on the front of the body. The presence of discoloration on the back of the body tended to reveal a deeper disorder. The "profile" position during treatment was particularly appreciated by the Egyptians. The patient would rest on one of his two sides, one leg slightly folded in front of him for comfort and his back turned to the therapist. The purpose of this position was to allow the placing of hands simultaneously in front of and behind the body.

Some organs, such as the liver and kidneys, are particularly receptive to such an energy approach. The therapist works either with both her palms or with the palm of one hand and three fingers united with the other hand (see *"c) Joining Three Fingers"* in Chapter VII, page 87).

When the person being treated has obvious emotional blockages, the simultaneous placing of hands on the front and back of the chakras will provide very good results.

5) Energy Cleansing

In order to prepare a person for the reading of his different auras, the Essenians developed a fairly complete method for cleaning one's "subtle identity card."

a) The Serpentine

Start with the dorsal side of your client (in prone position). The client lies on his or her belly. You can do this on both sides of the body (profile position) when you notice tightness or disorganized or polluted energy (for example, in the case of a smoker or someone with another kind of addiction). The Serpentine treatment when the patient is in the profile position involves the therapist's two hands placed in continuity, one and another, according to the following pictures. The therapist's breathing is free during the Serpentine.

This is an important treatment, more than you have likely imagined. The Serpentine was systematically reintroduced at the beginning of each healing session because of its harmonious impact.

For student-therapists not used to working with both hands, this exercise is also an excellent learning opportunity.

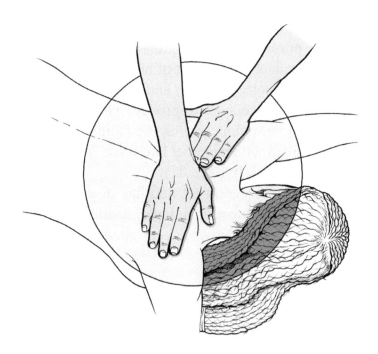

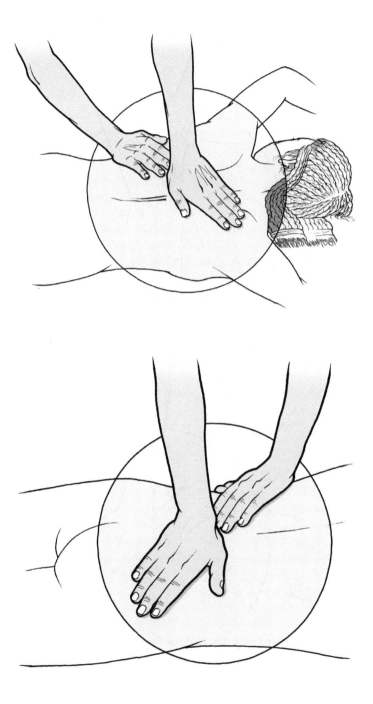

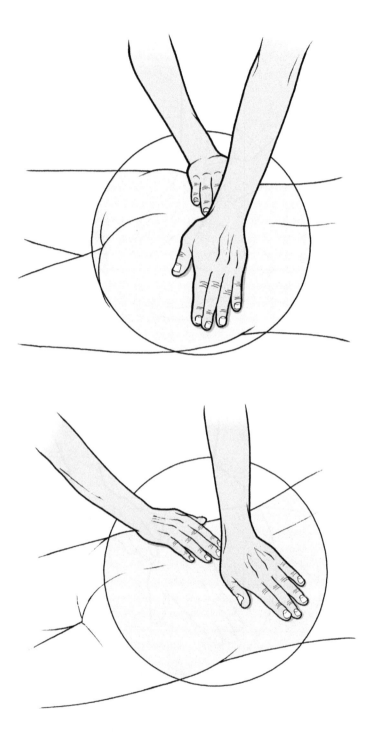

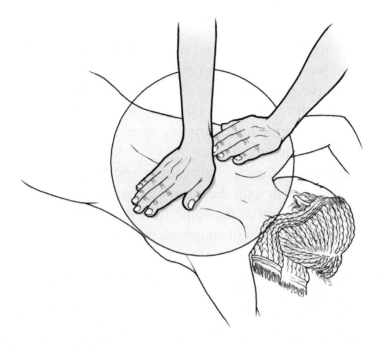

Complete this treatment by placing two hands at the top of the kidneys for a long time.[3]

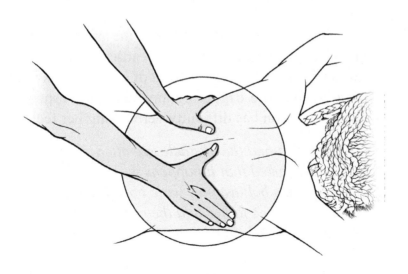

---

3   *The two hands are joined in a triangle shape on the area of the kidneys.*

b) The Stream

This method is performed on the front side of the client. Place the palm of your hand at the level of the pubis.[4] Very slowly, move your hand up along the client's body to the laryngeal chakra (the fifth chakra). While doing so, make very slight movements undulating from right to left and left to right, like a stream.

At the level of each chakra, stop and make a very slow, circular movement with the palm of your hand. The pressure needs to be firm but at the same time gentle. At the level of the throat, your hand will simply stand—that is, no movement or pressure. For greater comfort, pour a trickle of therapeutic oil along the vertical axis (from the base of the pubis to the throat) before starting this treatment.

It is not unusual for this treatment, when performed with all the required slowness, awareness, listening, and love, to provoke waves of emotion in clients.

The therapist must remain attentive to identify the precise area of the body, or chakra, that serves as a trigger for emotions, or perhaps even physical pain. The greatest attention, though, must be given to the impact of the hand on the laryngeal chakra.

The touch applied should be soft, because many emotional situations are concentrated in the form of energy knots in this area. It is best to avoid triggering any suffering, especially when a treated person has difficulty verbalizing her feelings.

> *"The effort and the obstacle are often so closely linked that it happens we can sometimes believe they were born for each other, one the father and the other one the mother, both help us to move forward."*[5]

---

4   *The bottom of the palm of the hand is placed delicately on the pubis bone.*
5   *La Demeure du Rayonnant (Home of the Radiant Sun) by Daniel Meurois).*

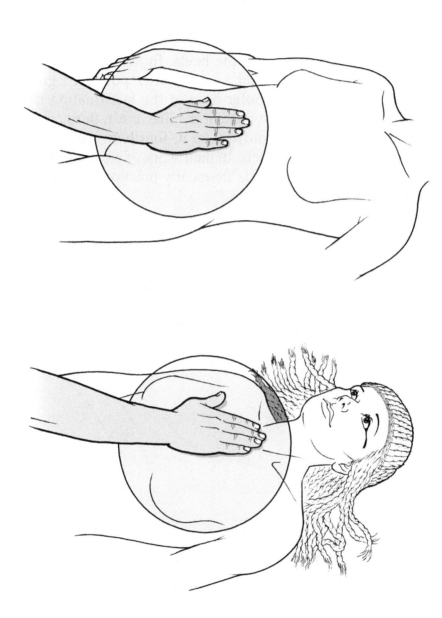

c) The Parallels

The Essenians called the two major nadis running along the right and left sides of the body "parallels." Each of these parallels starts from a "secondary chakra" on each shoulder and goes down the body to the heels. In the course of this route, they each encounter some energy points of great importance: first at the outer base of the last floating rib, second at the groin area, where at the iliac crest, third on the inside of the thigh and midway up it, fourth on the back of the knee, and lastly the heels. In their work of cleaning subtle bodies, the ancient therapists frequently practiced the etheric incision along these two nadis.[6]

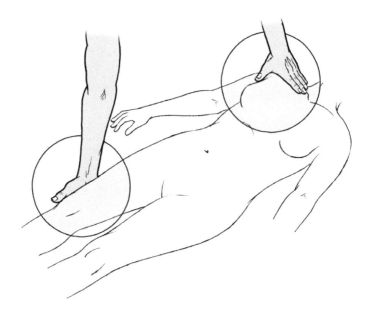

There was a second method for cleaning these parallel axes. This work (as shown in the picture above) consists of placing one hand at the energy center of the shoulder of a

---

6   *See p. 68, The Great Book of Essenian & Egyptian Therapies by Daniel Meurois & Marie Johanne Croteau.*

client and the other hand at the back of the knee. Next, the first hand is positioned on the last floating rib and the second on the iliac bone, as shown below.

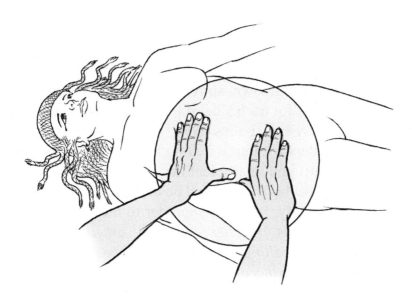

d) Sweeping

Here is a last technique. Sweeping was used to prepare for an aura reading, and to reduce any porosity of the "parallels," the two major nadis running along the right and left sides of the body.

Porosity is defined as an energy leakage identified during an etheric palpation or an aura reading. This phenomenon is much more common than most think. Because the causes are multiple and treatment must be determined on a case-by-case basis, it can be said that these energy leaks are at the origin of a great number of states of fragility, even if only one of the two sides of the body is involved. The method by itself is very simple. Its power lies in the energy bridge that must be created between the therapist and the client.

It should be noted that, during this process, it is very common for the one receiving the treatment to perceive an infinity of bubbles "sparkling" in him. The feeling of crystals bursting can also be felt strongly.

Generally, this is a sweet sensation, an astonishing feeling of the presence of peace that settles or is amplified in the client as soon as the treatment is completed.

Here is how to proceed. First, place your two hands side by side, palms facing down, above the client's shoulder. Here is how to proceed for each side of the body. First, place your two hands side by side, palms facing down, above one of the patient's shoulders without touching her. Slowly move your hands down until you finally feel her etheric body radiating. When this is done, both hands will be lowered slowly, side by side, along the body, from the shoulder to the knee. *(Before the treatment begins, the client should be asked to visualize a white veil gently rolling over the treated area at the rate of the movement of the therapist's hands.)*

It is also possible to practice this exercise in contact with the skin, as the Egyptians liked to do. Note that it is not uncommon for the person being treated to experience slight jolts, like small electrical discharges, when the therapist's hands reach the pelvic area. There is no need to worry about this. At the same time the subtle organism is cleaned, the scanning with both hands generates an energy supply, which is the basis of this reaction. One does not work here on the nadis but instead draws a veil of white light on the half of the body being focused on.

> *"We imagine The Soul is located at the heights of the being, but (...) it is always at the deepest of its valleys. Indeed in its caves is where we must look for it."[7]*

---

7   *La Demeure du Rayonnant (Home of the Radiant Sun) by Daniel Meurois).*

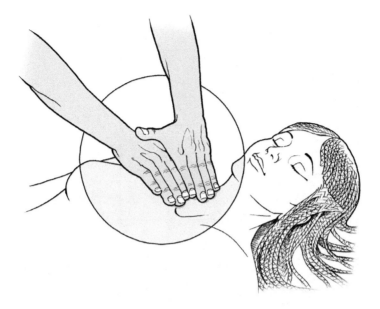

Chapter VII

At the Heart of a Technique

1) Intuitiveness and Precision

It is, a priori, quite unusual to associate the words "heart" and "technique." And yet this perspective, or rather this state of mind, is essential to putting into practice the methods described in this book.

To be at the heart of a technique is to be one with it. It is integrated to the point of losing the coldness of being "just" a technique.

Such an attitude, however, does not ignore rigor, and the practices of the ancient Egyptians and Essenians will probably appear difficult to truly grasp. Indeed, to feel from inside the language used by the soul and the body as well to open to the universal Wave of Healing and to retransmit this in the greatest transparency while remaining structured, precise, and down-to-earth is not an easy task.

Most of the difficulty lies, no doubt, in the delicate marriage of intuitiveness and technical precision. Intuitiveness speaks to inner listening, of letting go and trusting, while technical precision refers to a know-how gained through the mastery of gestures and specific knowledge.

These two characteristics of the energy transmitter that the therapist ideally represents are, alas, often perceived as antagonistic. However, the left and right brains should not be thought of as being in opposition to one another. Rather, there is a state of balance that can be achieved. We speak, in fact, of an art mixed with a science or a science with artistic elements.

With what my own perceptions have allowed me to bring back from the past, I have always been amazed at how much the hand movements of an Egyptian or Essenian therapist moving on a sick body evoked a dance—or, more precisely, a ballet. Precision and flexibility were, without context, the characteristics of their mastery.

Most of the gestures were performed with the therapist's eyes closed. His hands were so sensitive that the therapist could immediately spot, with a simple touch, the areas or points to be treated on a patient.

If you are seriously interested in the methods described here, I encourage you to work resolutely in this direction.

The grace of the movements, which might seem meaningless to some, develops on its own, as a real harmony unfolds in the practice of the therapist. In this sense, spontaneously while retaining a necessary simplicity, this is not an artifice but, on the contrary, a mark of real connection with the Divine. The development represents a natural extension of the sacred, which is always beautiful. As for the precision of the gestures with the positioning and movement of the hands, it does not induce the slightest rigidity. The ancients did not set up a rigid structure for the teaching of their practices and techniques.

Thus, the technical indications and methods described here are, above all, benchmarks. They are susceptible to variations or extensions insofar as the feelings and know-how of the therapist will bloom.

The therapist must integrate them enough to realize that they represent a kind of "grid of references," not bars of a jail.

Although it corresponds to a precise reality, for example, the path of a nadi will never be a continuous line not to be crossed.

The Egyptians understood that each human body, beyond its typical and classical functioning, has its own logic and balance. It is up to the therapist to learn how to decode it and help it express itself. Each body has its own levers of action. This awareness was certainly one of the fundamental elements of the therapeutic discipline as it was taught in the past. As such, any technical element serves as a basis for reflection and development for the one who puts it into practice without feeling compartmentalized. Offering a treatment such as taking a pill is laughable, as this would have no meaning behind it. I have been told that that is fine in some modalities, but still ....

2) Hands and Fingers

a) Hands Flat

In general, during treatments, hands should be employed with palms facing down. The most common mistake is spreading one's fingers apart to better cover an area. In doing so, the current of healing is dispersed. A quick reading of the auras of the hands will reveal this. Small kinds of luminous escapes similar to cigarette smoke will be visible between each finger, especially at the junction and articulation points. The radiance of the hand's energy extends by spreading but loses its concentration, which is not the therapist's goal during any treatment. Focusing a ray of healing was indeed at the heart of Egyptian therapeutic education.

The therapists of this period had noticed, after long observations, that the healing of a zone of the body is often initiated by the planting in it of a certain number of "luminous seeds." They understood that these "seeds" are born from the points of impact of a hand on an organ and that they grow gradually, ending up with luminous filaments between them. What results is similar to a network or threads whose intensity and activity restore health. In other words, a hand works by way of "infiltration." This is so effective because the hand is a vibrational whole, leaving no room for leaks or dispersion.

In Egypt, it was common to work simultaneously with both hands held flat, palms facing down, either one hand on one spot and the other a far distance away but still in relation (generally, the sick organ and its chakra director) or sandwiching a zone of the body between the palms (for example, one hand under the body at the level of a kidney and the other on the front of the body on the same kidney).

b) The Furrow

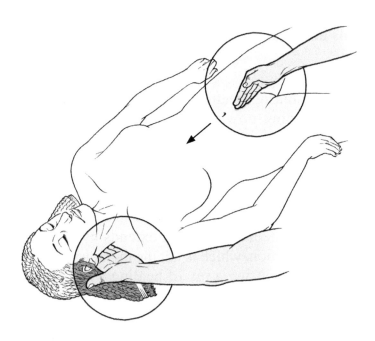

The Essenians liked work done with the edge of a hand. It was used like a plow to gently trace a furrow in the Ether of an organism. The furrow in question was "dug" very slightly and very slowly, without real pressure on the skin, usually from the bottom up, along a nadi. This technique can be performed with one hand while the other is in contact, on the opposite side of the body, with the point of arrival of the furrow.

This method is used to widen a circulation channel that's suspected to be weakened or fouled with etheric waste due to a series of emotional situations that have yet to be overcome. Such waste can be visualized in the form of small crystals of a grayish-yellow color, sometimes tinged with brown.

c) Joining Three Fingers

This method consists of joining three fingers (the thumb, index finger, and middle finger)[1] together in order to bring out a single ray of healing. It was extremely popular with the ancients. The thumb was associated with the overall strength of the uncreated, the index finger with the accuracy of the planet we now call Jupiter, and finally the middle finger with the great dissolvent that is time, Saturn. Anyone with some subtle perception ability knows how their beam of united light is capable of the precision of a scalpel.

Most of the difficulty lies, no doubt, in the delicate marriage of intuitiveness and technical precision. The ray of light aroused by the union of these three fingers extends with force over a distance of ten to fifteen centimeters (or four to six inches). It is up to each therapist to test their ability before beginning a treatment to ensure they stand the right distance away from their client's body. The ray must be employed on given area with still, precise, and slow movements.

In both cases, you can easily see the decongesting and very active power of the light beam that's created. It is not uncommon for the client to feel physically touched exactly where the ray is pointing. This feeling can sometimes be accompanied by pain. This is normal and will hurt no more than the burning sensation experienced when an alcohol-soaked pad is placed on a scratch to disinfect it.

---

1   *See p. 66, The Great Book of Essenian & Egyptian Therapies by Daniel Meurois & Marie Johanne Croteau.*

I must now note an extension of this method, which seems to have developed mainly from the Healing Temple of Abydos[2] in Egypt. I personally call this the "dropper" method.[3]

Once the three fingers are united, make a series of short squeezes (like squeezing a dropper). The ray of light projected onto the treated zone will be reinforced with each squeeze executed by the fingers. When one wants to relieve a point or release a precise area that's in severe pain, this method is particularly effective. It was used extensively on the gallbladder, kidneys, and bladder.

3) Preparation of the Area to Be Treated

The Egyptian and Essenian therapists attached great importance to disinfecting an area to be treated before starting an actual treatment. This disinfection did not apply to the whole body but rather to a part of it when a problem needed to be treated locally. It is a way to prepare an operative field.

The three-finger method previously described should be used. With the united ray of light that is created, draw on the body, from a distance, several series of vertical and horizontal lines so as to create a set of braces.

The zone that is drawn will be washed away with all the etheric dirt, and that area will become more open to the treatment shown below.

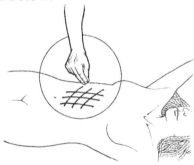

---

2   *https://en.wikipedia.org/wiki/Abydos,_Egypt.*

3   *See p. 67, The Great Book of Essenian & Egyptian Therapies by Daniel Meurois & Marie Johanne Croteau.*

4) Dynamization

a) The Cross of Life

This very simple technique involves areas that clearly appear to be suffering from energy loss. The Essenians, particularly concerned with the tone and quality of the voice, used it a lot in the region of the larynx to tone its chakra director. They had noticed that this area is among those that are most subject to significant energy fluctuations. Many emotions indeed come "rushing" through this space. Anger, fear, sadness, and a thousand other manifestations of the state of the soul meet there and leave traces behind most of the time, leading to the spot's weakening.

Always using the same joined three fingers, an Essenian therapist would draw crosses of life (ankhs) around the perimeter of the larynx region of a patient. Though they were circumscribing it, they were also dynamizing it harmoniously. The Egyptian cross of life symbolizes fertility and regeneration. The picture below shows the direction of the movements to be performed when using the three-finger method.

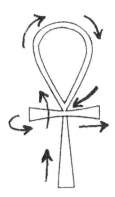

b) Seeding

Although less precise than the previous method, this practice is still worth mentioning because it allows work to be done efficiently and dynamically on larger and sometimes unclear areas of the body in the case of a difficult diagnosis. With the help of your hand, quickly grasp "in the air" a mass of light and project it energetically onto the body of the patient, almost like sowing seeds. This exercise should be repeated about ten times over the area that needs to be treated.

I am well aware of the strange, and even disconcerting, manner of this technique, as well as how it might make some people smile. Yet it must be understood that its effectiveness is conditioned by the relationship the therapist has with what is generally called pranic energy.

Indeed, here more than ever, the therapist must perceive the light as a tangible element and a force that belongs to him to project. This implies a state of being in which the therapist seeks particular modifications based on the vibrational state of his hands—their "etherization," you could say.

Such a state of consciousness is often manifested in the form of numbness in the hands and arms, which, strangely, removes none of their sensitivity to the subtle. If the therapist is in the required mind-set, he will clearly perceive the light as something he has a responsibility to "play" with.

5) Emotional Liberation

The liberation of the emotional charges of clients remained the constant concern of the Egyptian and Essenian therapists. They were aware that certain groups of cells and organs can easily memorize emotional states and then become sources of a multitude of disorders. As a result, the ancients believed it was essential to relieve a body and soul of disturbing emotions.

They favored the soft aspect of their therapeutic approach, even though it operated out of the consciousness of a client. It was possible, of course, for a given therapy to result in emotional outbursts from a patient when extreme tensions were brought to the point of causing the person a meltdown. Most of the time, however, the elimination of the emotions went smoothly.

90

Consequently, their practices tended to be performed with softness and were carried out in acceptance of the fact that sometimes a bit of time must pass before seeing results. They always preferred the depth of work done slowly to an energetic upheaval that can be difficult to control and likely to occur again.

Liberating a suffering being from pain—yes, that was the goal, but not at the cost of the person's destabilization elsewhere. In other words, it was important to not trigger emotional blockages. It is important to know how to do this with mastery—that is to say, with awareness and love. It is also important not to leave the patient "in a void" with what has manifested within her. In this sense, we can say that the softness, even the tenderness, of the Egyptian-Essenian practice represents a security in itself.

a) The Stream (2)

We will resume the exercise described in Chapter VI, page 76, as part of the energy cleansing of the body. It will suffice, however, to complete the work by placing the hands at the top of the patient's ribcage, with one hand positioned horizontally to join the clavicles and the other vertically on the sternum.

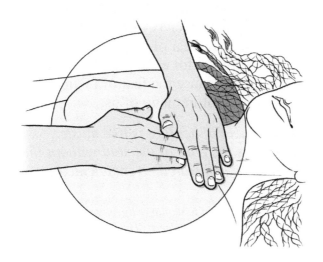

b) Method of the Diagonals

Those who have memorized the map of the major nadis[4] of the human body know that two major axes of energy meet in the center of the chest like a pair of straps. One extends from the left shoulder to the outer side of the last floating rib on the right-hand side of the body, and the other starts at the right shoulder and reaches down to the outer side of the last floating rib on the left-hand side. Together, they form a kind of big X whose two arms intersect at the heart chakra.

When performing this exercise, aim to place your hands in such way that they can follow the path of this X. The hand in the lower position should be placed slightly under the breast in order to cover the whole area of the lower ribs.

First, place one of your hands flat at the hollow of the right shoulder and move it gently to the heart chakra. Then move the other hand from the lower left to the heart chakra (Figure 1). In the second step, simply move the hand resting on the left side to the right (Figure 2). For the third and fourth steps, one will perform the same movements again but starting on opposite sides, so that the X of the nadis is totally covered by the whole exercise. If necessary, the therapist will change position relative to the patient for greater comfort in the practice.

This Method of the Diagonals is extremely effective when employed to release painful cellular memories due to a difficult relationship with society or life itself. These emotions are often connected to the fear of living and confronting others (anxiety when in a crowd, for example). In my opinion, this is an essential practice because the fear of facing life, or certain aspects of life, is present in many of us.

> *"The miracle of healing is like music.*
> *It touches the ears of the soul without the*
> *need to be translated or commented on."*[5]

---

4   *See p. 29, The Great Book of Essenian & Egyptian Therapies by D. Meurois.*
5   *Les Enseignements premiers du Christ (The Premier Teachings of the Christ) by Daniel Meurois.*

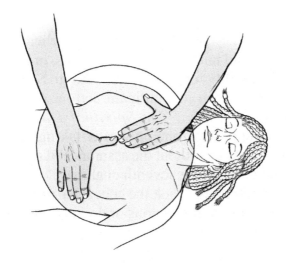

fig. 1

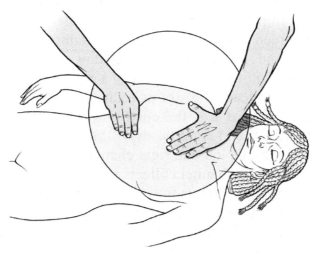

fig. 2

It is undeniably more important today than it was a few millennia ago. The Egyptians often preceded the Method of the Diagonals with harmonization work on the laryngeal chakra and ended by cleaning the bile duct with the help of the three united fingers.

c) The Coccygeal Memories

The coccyx is certainly one of the most delicate body parts to treat. Behind and under it—in other words, in direct contact with it—is the mighty force of the Kundalini. So touching the tailbone is far from an insignificant action. As I mentioned before (in chapter Five, *The Spiritual Dimension*), one should intervene in this zone only after taking the necessary precautions and never without the assurance of a good opening of the coronal chakra (the seventh chakra).

The ancient therapists took the coccygeal area into account in order to elicit liberating visions or dreams, especially when the person receiving treatment was feeling internally stuck in his life.

The relevant blockages can be of two kinds: a past burden dragged as a millstone in life making a patient "hit a ceiling" in their consciousness, or tension stemming from a physical symptom.

A real burden often is facing the uncertainty of the future. Life changes and risk-taking are slowed down or not options at all. The internal attitude is the source of a multitude of diseases.

In order to release the strains related to these two types of heavy weights, it was the custom to work with energy pulses on the left and right bases of the coccyx in order to get in touch with the left and right channels of the axis of the Kundalini. The left channel collects the baggage of the past, while the right concentrates the energy germs generated by a resistance to the future.

To perform the Egyptian technique, place your hands on the coccyx of the patient as shown in the figure below.

> *"Believing with confidence is very beautiful,*
> *being aware after having tasted is very*
> *interesting, but knowing for finally inviting*
> *the silence within is even greater."*[6]

---

6   *La Methode Du Maitre (The Method of The Master) by Daniel Meurois.*

94

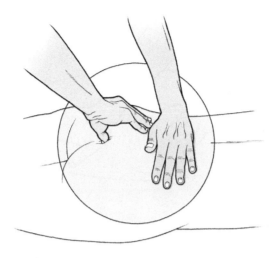

The thumb of the hand working to heal the coccyx will be positioned at the base of it, with a slight displacement to the right or left, depending on the channel being treated. The physical pressure applied must be very measured, with the main part of the treatment being carried out by the energy impulses (with help from the thumb). During this time, the other fingers of the same hand should be positioned on the sacred region. As for the second hand, place it very naturally, and horizontally, on the lumbar area of the body.

It frequently happens that a therapist must simultaneously treat the right and left channels of the Kundalini. In such a case, this should be done by positioning the thumb at the exact base of the coccyx and then slowly raising it to the sacred vertebrae area. Keep the pressure of the thumb very moderate, and be aware of the pain the client may experience. During this phase, the second hand is positioned as shown in the drawing below (Figure 1). Slowly move it back to the heart chakra at the same rate as you move the thumb toward the sacred region. The practice ends with the two hands aligned, one on the second chakra and the other on the fourth chakra (Figure 2).

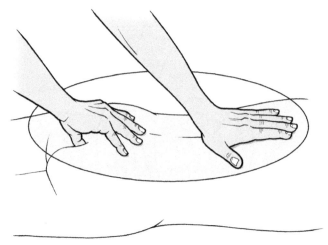

fig. 1

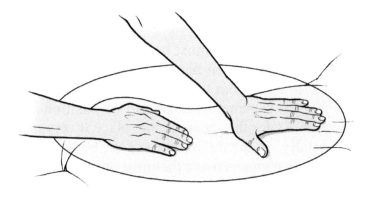

fig. 2

d) Neutralizing Stress

Although the notion of stress is relatively new in our modern world, the reality of it and its consequences existed a few millennia ago. The reasons for stress were different then, however, and it was less generalized, less pegged to daily life, which, though not easy, was not as hectic as it is today.

The priest-therapists had noticed that their therapies sometimes seemed to "slide" on some people. Such a patient appeared to be resistant to any energy intake or unable to be receptive to it. The priest-therapists attributed this to a kind of vibrational armor resulting from a mixture of physical fatigue, mental attitudes, and uncontrolled emotions. They also felt that this ended up creating a kind of memory or reflex, often leading the being to behave like a "piece of wood" in front of the contribution of a gentleness, such as a treatment. Their observations eventually led them to develop a short method to relax the armor built up by stress. Their goal was to make it, in a way, porous.

This method consists of interacting with the spleen and a specific point located on the inner and superior faces of the left breast, which is an energy stimulator of the thymus. This is how they proceeded at the beginning of a therapy session when they saw the need for it. With the help of the thumb, a therapist would practice slow massages clockwise on the area corresponding to the spleen on the left side of the body. From this area, still with the thumb, they went up along the sternum until they met the cardiac chakra. From there, they directed their thumb toward a precise point on the superior internal face of the left breast while also in direct contact with the skin.

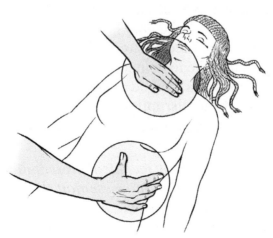

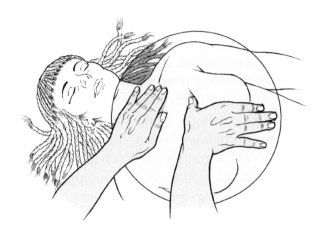

This whole gesture draws, as you can see, a sort of lunar crescent extending from the spleen to the reflex point of the thymus. Such a point is easy to identify because it is particularly sensitive to the pressure exerted by the thumb. This pressure should be accompanied by an extremely discreet circular movement, always in a clockwise direction.

It should be noted that some people cannot handle even the slightest touch of the therapist's thumb on this particular area. The pressure can indeed be excessively painful and sometimes unbearable. It should be introduced accordingly in a moderate way. Though such pressure and the pain it provokes are never pleasant for the patient, the goal is certainly not to make it a torment-generating source of stress!

Finally, I would like to point out that staying in tune to the pain and sensations this method causes a patient is extremely important here. If the disruption is too strong and lasts too long, this could cause discomfort to the patient.

Note: *At this point in my technical presentation, it should be noted that the Egyptian and Essenian therapists taught their students to regularly take the "moral pulse" of a person being treated. One cannot imagine a treatment worthy of the* *name without a therapist demonstrating his compassion for a patient through discrete and thoughtful physical contact.*

This contact is carried out with gentleness and by listening, with a hand placed simply on a wrist, under the back of the neck, or both at once. The loving human therapist must silence the learned technician within. The goal is quieting the rational mind.

May we find today fully the first sense—healthy, logical, and joyful.

Chapter VIII

The Therapist-Channel

Anyone who has studied the field of energy therapies even a little bit knows very well that being a therapist is a privileged path determined by the Universal Flow of Life to offer healing.

In the circles of what some call prâno-therapy, it is also obvious to affirm the following: "It is not me who heals."

There is certainly nothing to say against such a declaration. However, this saying can be overused and repeated without the necessary understanding of what it implies and requires from a therapist.

1) Channeling of What?

Being a channel during a treatment? Yes, of course. But channeling what? Let me be clear, though, at the risk of appearing prosaic: A channel is a conduit, a pipe of different calibers. Finally, it can be connected to a multitude of sources of varying clarity, some not even clear at all! Thus, though it is easy to call oneself a channel of a superior force, it is much less easy to be a real channel.

This fact is certainly not new. The priest-therapists of ancient Egypt and Mount Krmel[1] of the Essenians knew it

---

1   See Chapter IV, *The Way of the Essenes: Christ's Hidden Life Remembered.*

very well, as they strove constantly to guide their students toward harmony, lucidity, self-observation, and common sense, resulting in mastery. The idea of channeling was as popular as it is today, even in a therapeutic context.

Indeed, as soon as techniques are no longer experienced like an enforced grid of elements, something happens in the consciousness of the therapist that opens the door to phenomena, even to presences that we can give all kinds of names.

Nowadays, it is so-and-so or a notable figure who is sometimes announced as coming to heal through the hands of a therapist. Formerly, it was the underworld god Osiris; a great pharaoh already passed to the Kingdom of the Dead, such as Neter;[2] or a guardian angel of the Essenian fraternity. It doesn't matter who, it is still much more about vibrational principles than a particular personality.

Problems stem from the way in which the principles are captured, then oriented and offered. In other words, everything is dependent on the level of consciousness of the therapist. This level of awareness implies honesty, simplicity, letting go, and, of course, compassion. It is not invented with only goodwill. It is not attained either by attending a long series of seminars. The level is patiently discovered through the global experience of life and by audaciously traversing it without limits.

The initiatory mysteries of the past, as well as the traditional periods of "retreat in the desert," had no other function than testing a therapist. He had to first learn to know himself without artifice on the emotional and narcissistic levels. To channel a wave of healing, a healer (or other person) must overcome those two levels.

I said many years ago that initiation was nowadays occurring on the streets. This is probably more true than ever today because our souls and our bodies have no other choice

---

2   *Divinities that, according to the faith of the ancient Egyptians, inhabited all the realms of nature, comparable to the devas of the Hindu tradition.*

but to grow in contact with the extraordinarily diverse trials of our lives and the acceleration of their rhythm.

In continuing to be educated in private and understated buildings, we are increasingly facing ourselves and what we have assimilated in a world that is constantly changing.

This established fact is both a gift and a test. Our times and society offer us the rare opportunity to focus on who we are and what we really want. Between authenticity and cheating, venality and integrity, every latitude is given to us. Taking into account the sum of the requirements mentioned in this book, the therapist is surprisingly at the precise intersection of such an awareness. As long as he claims to have a certain perspective—that is, a real Service of Life—he is called to test himself regularly. Otherwise, he gets caught in his own reflection.

Lying to others is certainly quite simple. Deceiving ourselves also is very easy, because self-hypnosis is a common phenomenon. But in both cases, awakenings are difficult and painful. So it is better to not boast about channeling anything or anyone, better to not inflate a huge bubble that will eventually burst, if only in the heart of hearts.

The truth is that the simple and the fluid always end up having the last word. The body and soul of the therapist are called to surrender to them.

2) Empowerment of the Hands

The empowerment of the hands is a phenomenon that can be expected, one day or another, by anyone in a state of communion with a Superior Principle. It usually manifests itself in a very spontaneous way through progressive loss of control of the hands. This loss of control is either partial and brief or complete and continuous during a treatment.

In both cases, it is the result of surrender, transparency, and trust on the part of the therapist.

The teachers of the Essenian fraternity affirmed that a therapist should neither seek it out nor flee its appearance. It imposes itself as an existing situation at a given moment during a practice. It was clear to the Essenians, however, that its absence was by no means a mark of internal elevation. In the practice of an art, there are multiple tools. None are superior to others, since each translates different sensitivities.

The phenomenon starts most of the time with a feeling of numbness in the hands. This numbness is due to a more or less significant release of their etheric counterpart. In other words, the ethereal mold of the hands is gradually extracted from its flesh form, resulting in the loosening of the personality of the therapist.

How are the hands moving in order to offer the treatment? The movements are performed with help from two forces. These forces are made up of different but convergent natures.

a) The Force of Transmission

The force of transmission results from the action of the Superior Consciousness of the therapist—that is to say, from the "zone" of his being that's beyond his incarnated personality but begins to manifest itself through the eighth chakra (see #5 in Chapter III, page 33). In such a case, the etheric body around the hands is only partially relieved, and the sensation of numbness remains slight. The therapist's hands are thus simply guided by a principle that acts as a bridge between the human and the supra-human.

In almost all cases, the manifestation of this phenomenon of transmission requires the therapist to have his eyes closed. The treatment is no more than an absolute meditation to such an extent that all the basic technical elements described in this book vanish for the therapist, who moves on to a higher awareness.

Just to be clear, the connection with this realm is very precise and not based on a belief system that leads to a typically vague intuition. There is, in fact, a surrender to a

Supreme Presence that is aware and knows and can remove any preconceptions as needed.

b) The Force of Channeling

The force of channeling is the real intervention of a Presence totally external to a therapist. It is manifested either by a complete numbness of the therapist's hands and arms, escaping his control, or by the presence taking possession of his whole body.

The therapist is, therefore, at this time overshadowed by the luminous presence that offers the therapy in his place. In such a case, we speak of channeling or even a trance since the body of the therapist is an instrument of a power that is beyond him and uses him in a sacred way. The therapist's consciousness is absent, absorbed by another universe of which he generally keeps no memories when he reintegrates into his body.

This phenomenon is much more rare than one might think and can present itself in a multitude of variants. It depends on the level of internal preparation of a therapist's level and his personal capacity to withstand the corresponding vibrational shock.

It is obvious that no therapist can decide on his own to treat a patient in this way. The phenomenon imposes itself, or it does not. It never results from a choice but rather from a state of the therapist's own person, which predisposes him to this type of service.

Is it even necessary, then, to specify that the quality of the enlightenment, and therefore of the presence that manifests itself, hinges solely on the therapist's purity of soul, his psychic equilibrium, and his physical resistance?

Those who, in ancient Egypt, showed such gifts in the practice of the therapies during the probationary period were severely controlled by the priest-therapists who trained them. The priest-therapists did not marvel at such a phenomenon, but it was considered extremely sacred, which is different.

105

They tried to extract from it any emotional context in order to approach it in an intimate, deep, noble, and luminous way.

During this kind of "therapeutic event," there is indeed a marrying of the universes. These merge within the body of the one who treats and whose vibrational rate increases considerably. The voice of the therapist can then change the therapist's behavior. As the therapist is not the one directing the vehicle, this is logical.

Finally, it should be noted that a client must be, in advance, informed of the possibility of such a manifestation during a treatment. Not everyone is receptive to this type of phenomenon and design of an energy treatment, nor is everyone comfortable with a subtle intervention as tangible and powerful as this one can be.

What seemed normal and obvious a few millennia ago is much less so today in our society. Still, though, a healing session always involves respect for the sensitivity and level of openness of the client. So, anything that could be beyond her ability to understand or imposed on her must be systematically removed.

In addressing this particular area of the energy therapies, I am well aware of my opening a huge parentheses of sorts, which is access to many metaphysical reflections. My intention is to not deal with them more extensively in these pages. However, it seems important to mention the topic because therapists as much as clients can be confronted with and deprived of this.

3) The Development of the Frontal Chakra

As part of the blossoming of the state of a therapist, the Egyptians and Essenians used to test themselves in self-control. It involved a priest-therapist observing his own frontal chakra (the sixth chakra). The way in which this inner-vision chakra appeared to him invited him to not lie to himself and thus played the role of regulator when faced with the possible derailment of his personality.

The Master Jesus Himself frequently recommended to his closest disciples, whether therapists or not, the analysis of this center, which he saw as an indicator of "the transparency of the conscience."

In His teachings on this subject, He distinguished three major levels in the development of the frontal center ("*Ajna*"). According to His words, it was up to each person to know where he was in the present instant and to strive to obtain a clear vision in certain moments of meditation.

a) Phase 1

At this first level of its development, the frontal chakra appears as a golden ring between the eyebrows when both eyes are closed and a real relaxation has settled in. This ring indicates a level of consciousness still gripped too much by the emotional world, which, to tell the truth, is not ideal when one embarks on the path of the therapies.

b) Phase 2

The second level of manifestation of this "third eye" appears as a very beautiful blue disc. The quality of the blue can be intense and deep, but this depends on the purity of the prana circulating in the network of nadis.

The appearance of the blue disc, which can be described as a more or less visible point that increases in size over time, indicates that the being is trying to calm his mental dimension.

He is beginning to possibly be able to gain altitude in relation to the multitude of events in life.

c) Phase 3

Finally, the third level of expression of the frontal chakra makes it appear in the form of a luminous star with five branches, though it is not possible to say whether it is moon-colored or sun-colored. The number five, which characterizes this star, necessarily brings us back to the quintessence of a being and speaks to the ability to understand beyond the contingencies of matter and time as conventionally perceived. This is why such a star indicates the possibility of access to the world of causes, including the Akashic Visions.

Master Jesus also taught that there are intermediate phases in the stages of development of the frontal chakra, especially between that of the blue disc and the five-pointed star. Various geometrical shapes, or even "white screens," can spring up and persist for long periods.

There is, however, a major point on which He insisted: The manifestation of the different stages of radiation of the frontal chakra must exclude any spirit of challenge, competition, or internal struggle. It would be stupid indeed to say to oneself, "I am only at this level. It is necessary that in so many months or years I will have passed to the next." Such a state of mind is incompatible with the harmonious development of the consciousness and the intimate necessities of its maturation. It is also important to understand that these levels of manifestation of the center *Ajna* do not necessarily have anything to do with the greatness of the soul of a being (i.e., his capacity to love and serve a luminous cause). They are in no way the barometer of what is often simplistically called the "degree of spirituality" of a person. A psychic center may well be constrained at some point in the history and evolution of a being so that other abilities can be cultivated and developed.

So let's not judge anyone, and don't discourage yourself, or even feel guilty, if your sixth chakra does not come in the form you'd like. The Akashic Records mention some meetings of Master Jesus and his close disciples. They asked him to teach them techniques for the development of the sixth chakra in order to "better read the souls of others and help them accordingly." It would be wrong to say that no method was communicated to them in this regard. However, I will not dwell on the description because it does not differ from what is still accessible today through disciplines like Kriya Yoga, or the yoga of purification. Such methods are therefore available to all those who are interested.

I prefer to evoke once again the very root of Christ's teaching. I am referring, of course, to the total and unconditional call to a Presence of Love transcending all the "technical" aspects of life that often imprison a being in their net. This does not mean "Long live ignorance and welcome only intuition!" Rather, it's "Let your heart be the ultimate conductor."

One's energy center is comparable to a musical instrument that is able to translate a certain melodic line. No one line is allowed to impose its melody on the whole score or hold the baton of the maestro.

Pharaoh Akhenaten once told his relatives that during all the years of learning at the Holy Mysteries, he imagined that the sixth chakra would finally appear to the meditator in the form of the eye or "oudjat," also called the Eye of Horus. He did not know then that this hieroglyphic representation would not correspond to the inner reality eventually encountered by him. Strangely, all the priests in charge of his training had failed to teach him about this, perhaps thinking that as future master of Egypt and "incarnated divinity" he possessed from the outset this basic knowledge.

According to Akhenaten, the realization occurred barely a week before he passed one of the major initiations. The awareness was cruel, all the more so because he did not dare to talk about it.

Keeping quiet about his anguish, the young prince submitted himself to the initiatory trial that his instructors had prepared for him. He said that, one night in the cave where he was kept for three days, something in him suddenly dissolved, allowing him to overcome his apprehension. He decided to abandon any desire to perceive the Door of Infinite Light that had been promised to him in the center of his skull and simply

109

rely on the crystal of his heart (or "seed cell," the holiest of the holies according to the Egyptians).[3]

If love lived there (as he'd been taught), if the abandonment of all fear was his liberator, and if the offering of one's being was his absolute motor, then the hopeful Door of Light would manifest itself there, in a form chosen by the Divine.

And, according to Akhenaten, the following happened: His consciousness experienced an expansion hitherto unparalleled, propelling him despite his young age to the threshold of mastery. Finally, in concluding his story, the pharaoh confessed that, even after this dazzling experience, he still could not access the proper perception of his frontal chakra because he could not get rid of the imprint of the Eye of Horus. "And what did you do?" asked one of his relatives. "Nothing. And I do not care," he answered coldly.

---

3   *See p. 23, The Great Book of Essenian & Egyptian Therapies by Daniel Meurois & Marie Johanne Croteau.*

Part Three

Chapter IX

An Aspect of Egyptian Heritage:
Perspectives on Body Image

1) The Sacred Square

The following information will probably surprise many of you. To my knowledge, it does not appear in any manuscript to date. And for good reason, as it has been transmitted orally. It is a system of references, forgotten today, that was once proven. This is probably the reason why the Akashic Memory allowed me to reconstitute it, at least in a broad outline.

The system was organized at the beginning of the reign of Amenhotep III, father of Akenaten. It continued to be used during the reign of Aï[1] until the clergy of Amun again imposed their laws and principles in all areas of life.

It reveals the existence of a sacred square, a kind of body diagram that therapists liked to use as a base. The basic image is of a human body divided into four zones determined by the meeting of symbolic vertical and horizontal lines.

---

1   *https://en.wikipedia.org/wiki/Ay.*

The point of intersection of these two lines was at the level of the heart, making the heart the master of the game.

According to the understanding of the therapists of the time, it is from the strength that this point represents, both in terms of density and in the universe of the subtle, that the harmony of a being is built.

By virtue of this principle, an ideal treatment is therefore organized (if possible) at the level of the heart and follows a kind of itinerary with its own logic, enabling a reharmonization of the body, organ after organ. When traced on the body, this route is a kind of "healing line" that evokes, as a whole, the route of the lemniscate, or infinity symbol.

In more precise terms, the healing wave is initiated at the center of the chest. It is lowered to the right zone of the abdomen, then brought to the right side of the rib cage, then moved down to the left abdomen, then drawn up along the left side of the chest, and finally shifted back to its starting point, the heart chakra. Such a vibrational course was followed by the ancient therapist's hands whenever a patient was suffering from troubles that were difficult to determine, when he was in a state of great fatigue, or when a disease was desynchronizing all his systems. So we can speak here of a real protocol, one that can be considered nowadays for treating diseases such as fibromyalgia (chronic fatigue), multiple sclerosis, and cancer. It encompasses the whole body while putting it in relation, organ after organ, with the present and past. It creates a multidimensional reality in which all the elements are closely linked to each other and express themselves as much in the concrete world as in the symbolic and spiritual dimensions.

To be well assimilated, it certainly merits being meditated on. In my opinion, it is not a matter of learning it by heart but of respecting the data in a rigid way. The diagram below proposes above all a "global navigation method" within the human body, as well as reference elements on which a therapist can rely when undertaking an overall treatment and a reflection.

According to this vision of the human body, each zone, with its organs, represents in its own way of an aspect of being as well as a level(s) of the implantation of suffering.

Treating one zone of the sacred square more than another is to bring the being into a relationship with the concrete, symbolic, and spiritual dimensions of it. Precise doors open to a Wave of Healing. Conversely, treating all four areas, keeping in mind the Egyptian design, brings a sense of total peace to the patient, dispelling the boundaries between his different levels of reality.

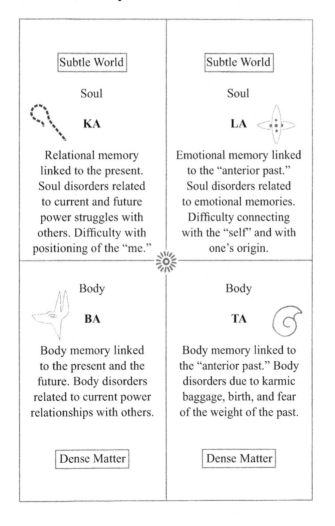

As you'll notice, each of the areas determined by the cross is supported by a great symbol evoking one of the four kingdoms of nature: mineral, vegetal, animal, and human. Each symbol connects to an archetype and a specific healing power. The priest-therapists visualized one after the other, according to the part of the body being treated—that is, according to the level of the being they were trying to touch.

The jackal is associated with the lower right part of the body, the crozier of power with the upper right part, the shell (ammonite) with the left inferior zone, and the hibiscus flower with the left thoracic region.

The letters appearing next to a symbol were internally pronounced repetitively, like a mantra, during each visualization phase. As for the central sun, which illuminates and orders the sacred square diagram, it obviously represents the Uncreated, the Source of All Life, the Divine Seed that animates the being. At the end of the treatment, the priest-therapist placed his hand on the heart chakra for a long time to anchor a Wave of Healing to impregnate the seed cell (which also refers to the deep memory of the patient, his "central bank of data," according to today's terminology).

It was common, at this precise stage of the treatment, for the priest to internally recite his own personal prayer. Each therapist was, in fact, bound to invent a prayer of therapy, a kind of invocation reserved for himself, that ultimately would revitalize all the work of healing undertaken.

It is important to note that this prayer should include thanks addressed to the Source of All Life since, in the end, it is She who acts.

> *"The key is to be a river by accepting that water is flowing through yourself."*[2]

---

2   *La Demeure du Rayonnant (Home of the Radiant Sun) by Daniel Meurois.*

2) The Point-Life

The notion of the seed-atom that was just mentioned was particularly venerated by the Egyptians. They called it the "point-life."[3]

In a way that might seem simplistic today, they believed that a human being was able to "think" from any vital area of the body, such as the intestine, the liver, or the stomach, for example. They placed the heart at the center of this conception and made it the seat of a specific thought as well as the door of access to a memory related to the origins of the being.

To let one's heart speak—to refer to one's deep knowledge—did not, for them, represent an attitude linked to vague intuition or a temporary emotional state. The heart connection expressed the sum of past experiences as well as their consequences printed in the body up to the present time.

This point-life or seed-atom therefore represented the confluence of a priest-therapist's concerns during each of the therapies he provided. The priest-therapist was hoping to "touch" the seed-atom, wash it if he felt it necessary, and then "load it" with a constructive memory. Although they were aware that the reality of this point is of a subtle nature—ethereal and astral—the priest-therapists felt its exact counterpart is in the dense matter of the body (hence their conviction that there is a real "brain" gifted with memory in the heart).

The students were taught that this precise point consists of forty crystals that, like diamond doors, sum up a being in his wholeness and give access to his depths—past, present, and future reunited.

It could be said that all this is just a fantasy, but do not forget that every cardiology surgeon today knows there is

---

3   *See p. 20, Les Maladies Karmiques (The Karmic Diseases) by Daniel Meurois-Givaudan. See also p. 25, The Great Book of Essenian & Egyptian Therapies by Daniel Meurois & Marie Johanne Croteau.*

an extremely precise point that must be avoided during open heart surgery. This point, if touched, causes instantaneous death, like cutting the cord connecting a patient's soul to his body or touching something so high and sacred that the body reality cannot bear the vibrational shock.

Amazingly, the HeartMath Institute[4] has highlighted the existence of a true "brain zone" in the heart. This fractional point consists of forty thousand cells. The activation of the cardiac rhythm starts there when a human being is conceived in the maternal womb, even before the brain's formation.

How can one not see a connection between this "mini nervous zone" from which springs the pulse of life and the traditional Egyptian "point-life"? It's also impossible not to consider the forty crystals of the priest-therapists and the forty thousand cells of this vital point newly brought to light.

3) Harmonization Symbols

a) Visualization

Regarding a global treatment linked to a serious illness or a profound disorder of the being, the ancient therapists first hoped to be able to heal by leaving an imprint within the seed-atom or point-life. To do this, beyond what they were trying to transmit through their hands, they placed significant importance on the harmonization symbols associated with the four major areas of the body, as previously described. In trying to reproduce their effects today, it is not enough to say that they visualized them internally. You have to know how these visualizations were practiced. During the initial phase, a therapist took three or four slow and long breaths in and out while being "cross-eyed" internally, so as to stimulate the frontal chakra area. He next released the pressure between the two eyes to hold his breath, lungs full. In the third phase, he

---

4   *https://www.heartmath.com.*

released the air through his nose by scraping the nasal cavity. And finally, he let come to him, behind his closed eyelids, the image of the symbol called. The notion of "Let it come" was crucial in the approach of the visualization because, for the priest-therapists, it was in no way a work of will.

The desired image would emerge internally, without the least bit of tension, as if progressively rising from the depths of a lake to the surface. In general, an Egyptian priest-therapist in Akhenaten's time completed his visualization practices by raising his consciousness to the top of his head while his hand rested on a patient's heart center. Once his consciousness was well placed at the level of his seventh chakra, he called on the image of a hand of light to be attached to him. In order to touch the point-life, he went so far as to feel the caress in a state of openness and communion, with the wave prolonged first through his body, then his arm, and finally his hand to the patient's heart.

b) Organs

In the same way they associated symbols with the four great areas of the body, the Egyptian priest-therapists of Akhenaten also linked each organ to an image with an archetypal value.

When they treated a specific organ, no matter the disorder a patient was suffering from, it was not unusual for them to use one of these images internally as an additional vector of action for healing.

I advise doing this only when one is already very familiar with all of the practices of the hands as described—that is, when the hand movements can be carried out with fluidity. because noncompliance can lead to an overload or congestion of the mind of the therapist during a healing session. The same recommendation was made three thousand five hundred years ago.

Here are the symbols that were most commonly used. Some refer to hieroglyphics, while others simply resemble organs.

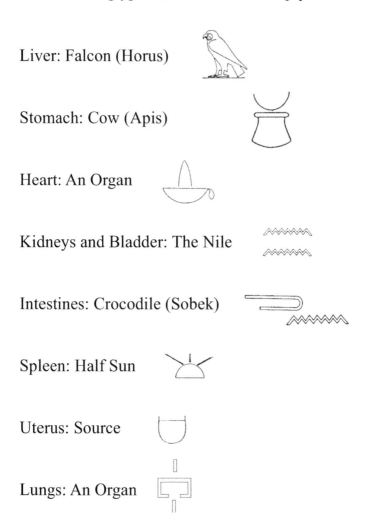

Liver: Falcon (Horus)

Stomach: Cow (Apis)

Heart: An Organ

Kidneys and Bladder: The Nile

Intestines: Crocodile (Sobek)

Spleen: Half Sun

Uterus: Source

Lungs: An Organ

4) The Rise of Consciousness

As I mentioned earlier (in Chapter Five), the evolution of a patient's consciousness was at the center of a priest-therapist's concerns, as much for the Essenians as for the Egyptians. The healing of the body could only be completed when the soul entered into a necessary mutation, meaning the patient's will was to purify himself and brush away the disease from within. No opportunity was missed by a priest-therapist to change what is now called the "vibrational level" of a person if she was fully aware of the metamorphosis happening within herself.

Because of the importance of the soul evolution, there was an emphasis on the cleansing of the major energy axis, causing the free flow of the vital force concentrated at the base of the spine. It is worthwhile to address this point once more in this book, in order to provide some additional insights into the conception that the ancients had of what is traditionally known as the ascension of the Kundalini.

As in the Eastern conception, the therapists I'm referring to spoke of a subtle triple channel that allowed the "Fire of Life" to ascend along the spinal cord. They assumed that the fusion of the right and left channels of the dorsal axis allowed the central channel to expand so that the force unfolded totally and powerfully, from the base of the being to the top.

The left channel (*Ida* in Sanskrit) was, according to them, traveled by a breath (*apana*). This breath was compared to rain, meaning a force going from top to bottom. The right channel (*Pingala*) was likened to dew. Its breath (*prana*) was perceived as going from the bottom to the top (i.e., offering the soil moisture to the sky).

The Egyptians and Essenians claimed that *apana* and *prana* responded to each other and maintained an energy motor. Nowadays, this is comparable to a battery with its two poles. They thought that the two channels, the *Ida and Pingala* (that we today think of as primary), resembled two vertical axes located on either side of the central channel (*Sushumna*) of the still embryonic Kundalini.[5] According to them, it is only with the progressive elevation of the consciousness that the *Ida and Pingala* begin to undulate under the stimulatory

---

5   *See p. 31, The Great Book of Essenian & Egyptian Therapies by Daniel Meurois & Marie Johanne Croteau.*

action of the *apana* and *prana*. Over the course of lives, the wave becomes such that the two axes eventually cross each other and create the ideal pattern found in all the traditional teachings of the subtle anatomy.[6]

When the crisscrossing becomes effective, the central channel (*Sushumna*) until then almost nonexistent, begins to expand and become active to constitute the royal road for the rise of the Kundalini. Dilated to the extreme, it appears to form just one pathway.

Analogously, it is the same principle that is implemented during the mastery of some Tibetan songs: two columns of air, one ascending and the other descending cross in the back of the throat of a lama, enabling an uninterrupted sound to be emitted for a very long time.

It goes without saying that when a person arrives at the fusion, and therefore at the smooth running of the Kundalini triple fire, the overall health of her being is realized. This does not mean that, during her incarnated life, the person in question will no longer be affected by difficulty, as dense matter imposes certain constraints. It means that the obstacles encountered will be sublimated, mastered, and used constructively as part of a *mission of Service*.

The being then becomes a true universal battery, reconciling in a single pacifying force the positive and the negative, the solar and the lunar, the fire and the water, the masculine and the feminine.

This state constitutes total mastery. The being has reached the state of Christlike or Buddhist realization. This does not mean that she must play the role of a Christ or Buddha in a historical way but that she ceases to be subject to the cycle of reincarnation.

With this perspective, great missionaries such as Master Jesus and Pharaoh Akhenaten taught the principles of health.

---

6   For an image of the caduceus used as a medical symbol, see
    https://en.wikipedia.org/wiki/Caduceus_as_a_symbol_of_medicine.

For them, being healthy did not just mean getting a healthy body. It meant not hiding "time bombs" deep inside, feeding nothing perverse in the cellars and attics of the heart. This meant having the body, soul and spirit be "layered" without the slightest dissonance. It meant being simply and happily one with the One.

May this book of perennial memories inspire this in our present.

ANNEX
The Method of the Master

Purification of the Eight Chakras

The purification of the Eight Chakras was taught directly by Master Jesus—Jesus Christ—to his disciples.[1]

Purification of the First Chakra

Introduction of *The Teaching of the First Chakra* according to Master Jesus

The base chakra—*Muladhara* in Sanskrit—was *Malkut* in the Kabbalistic Tradition. It was the Kingdom of Mother Earth, the point of reference, the foundation that no one could do without, in order to begin their path of Realization.

According to Christ, this Kingdom took the appearance of an immense cave, rich in endless gems and precious stones. These were proclaimers of the Diamond of consciousness located at the upper extremity of the being. Master Jesus encouraged us to regularly visualize this cave like a geode. According to Him, each of the crystallizations constituting this geode existed in energy and corresponded to a potential of creation—potential which every human body had acquired over time and which constituted a kind of memory of the faculties of the human species.

---

1   *"La Methode du Maitre" (Method of the Master) by Daniel Meurois.*

He recommended to practice this visualization standing with our feet firmly planted on the ground, as well as sitting in the classic meditation position. Why standing? Because He taught us that the soles of the feet were in direct connection with the first chakra.

> *As Above So Below, As Below So Above*
> — Hermes Trismegistus

This means that the energy residing at the very base of the human body is just as respectable as the energy manifesting at the top of the skull. When Master Jesus spoke "in altitude" of the first chakra, He was rehabilitating it by telling us how the first chakra's strength touched the Heavens while staying connected with the Earth Element.

- Place both hands on your knees, palms down.

- Pay attention to the base of your body and try to feel roots digging into the ground, just as if you were a tree. Maintain this inner attitude as you try to perceive a kind of gravity, accompanied by the sensation of sinking into the ground, or at least becoming one with it.

- Now bring your attention above your head and feel the presence of a beautiful ball of white light. Invite it to slowly descend into you until it floods your base chakra.

- Breathe in peacefully through the nose while visualizing the winding of a luminous spiral at the base of your body. Roll out this coil while exhaling. (Note that the arrow in Figure 1 below indicates the direction of this progression.)

Practice seven inhalations/exhalations of this type, breathing freely between each.

126

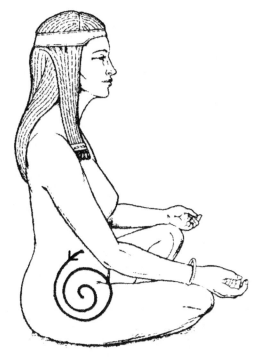

fig. 1

Purification of the Second Chakra

*Introduction of **The Teaching of the Second Chakra** according to Master Jesus*

The second chakra—*Svadisthana* in Sanskrit and *Iesod* in the Kabbalistic Tradition—associated with the Water Element, was considered especially sacred. Situated one hand below the navel, Master Jesus insisted on the sacredness of this chakra to be the true portal of the Incarnated Human Temple while expressing the human foundations.

Its mastery was essential, He affirmed, because it is the place of a natural antagonism. An antagonism not between Above and Below, but between the Forces of Aggregation and Dispersion which characterize the mechanism of life in general.

As an example, He mentioned the most basic biological function linked to the second chakra; the elimination of urine. To His understanding, the body didn't get rid of the urine as an impure matter but produced a substance of which the components were part of the Equilibrium of the entire Nature.

Further the semen liquids produced by the body were not impure at all and entered in a mystical approach for Him: *"If you hear me, then you understand that I am the Semen of my Father while you are the Matrix that receives It. I am the Threshold and the Foundation of the Temple just as much as the One who guides you between its pillars."*

- Place your left hand on your left knee, palm down, while your right hand is positioned on your second chakra.

The goal of this position is to generate a specific energy circuit with the left knee—the Entrance of the Temple Itself—which is associated to the Moon symbolizing the emotional and intuitive nature of the human.

Master Jesus recommended to visualize a crescent moon in the palm of our left hand sitting on our left knee. When done, we should feel the current of energy starting to flow from this moon to our heart, and then from our heart to our second chakra, before returning to its starting point, the lunar crescent.

He advised us not to move on to the next phase of the exercise until after we had internally followed the current of life in this energy loop at least three to four times in a row. According to Him, this preparatory phase promotes the regulation and drive of sexual energy. It makes the base of this subtle channel less porous, which the Traditions call *Ida*, and which is one of the three branches of the ascensional force of the Kundalini.

He spoke of *Ida*[2] like a river whose bed sometimes tended to present a thousand small breaches near its source, breaches which made it disperse and carry alluvium, animal instincts drawn from Ether.

He ended His discussion on this energy channel, *Ida*, and told us that the position is reversed in women. Ideally, women[3] should therefore put their right hand on their right knee and their left hand on their second chakra when practicing this exercise. However, according to Him, failure to respect this position had no harmful effect on the organism

---

2   *See p. 31, The Great Book of Essenian & Egyptian Therapies by Daniel Meurois & Marie Johanne Croteau.*
3   *The same goes for the channel named Pingala counterpart of Ida. Pingala initializes on the left side of the dorsal axis of women.*

and consciousness. This only resulted in an absence of intervention on the drive side of the woman.

- Let your consciousness descend from your back to the base of your body by perceiving a white sun there. Bring it up to your second chakra with a short breath in.

When we were asked to place our consciousness at a specific point in the body, it did not mean focusing our attention on the area in question. For that would have been equivalent to an approach of the mind observing from the outside a body area.

It is therefore a question of identifying as much as possible with the specific presence of the energy of life—the white sun—in which the top of our skull is bathed. It is about placing our consciousness in this source point as if the totality, of what we are able to perceive of ourselves, inhabits it. The secret of this centering and of this particular perception of oneself is discovered quite naturally in the relaxation and surrender to the Divine in oneself.

It is very common for small tickles to be felt at the top of the head during this phase of the exercise. These reflect a movement of activation of the seventh chakra. There is no need to linger there but to enter into an even deeper relaxation, which will spontaneously bring our consciousness to descend with tenderness and slowness along our spine.

Master Jesus insisted that for this descent to be perfect, it did not have to be decided mentally. It is not because one judges that "it must be the moment," but because it is recognized that it cannot be otherwise. There is a logical and loving call from our consciousness that goes down and is recognized by our body.

Although this descent is like a fire, Rabbi Jesus compared it to a powerful—albeit very gentle—water current descending from the heights of a mountain to irrigate the valley. This is how He explained the reason for the sensation of freshness which generally accompanies the descent of the "Fire of Consciousness" all along the back.

- Then, bring this sun down to the base chakra with a short breath out.

- Ideally, repeat four sets of seven inhalations/exhalations. Between each set, take care to observe a deep silence and focus your attention on your second chakra.

When the presence of the white sun is down the base chakra, breath in to bring up this sun to the second chakra, then breath out to bring it down to the first chakra. Breathing needs to be brief and relaxed. The white energy fire will circulate twenty-eight times between the first and second chakra, which is a lunar and aquatic number to meditate on.

Note that with each breath in and out, the air should gently scrape the back of the nasal cavity, causing a slight noise.

Purification of the Third Chakra

Introduction of *The Teaching of the Third Chakra* according to Master Jesus

"You will know, my friends, that there are generally two ways of being in this world .... The first way is the one of the man-animal, feeling the imperative need "to mark their territory." This way of being manifests itself on all levels. The physical level is, of course, the first concern. Strength and narcissistic beauty have only one goal of spreading out in the eyes of the world. This level is in close correspondence with the second, that of emotions, in full effervescence, which eventually leads to a large number of verbal and cerebral outbursts. I will tell you that this way of being is that of fighting and the search for success.

The second way is the one of humans who understood to be at the state of confidence as well as trusting the correctness of what Life places in their path. Those ones know that they do not need ramparts nor weapons or shields to protect anything since the whole universe is offered to them as an inheritance.

Why would they leave their marks in the four corners of a field as soon as they understood Infinity is their means of expression? This way of being characterized those who have exceeded the drive for triumph. They are the ones who look towards this true glory which is Splendor. What is there to conquer and to want to constantly affirm when everything belongs to us from all eternity? Splendor is the embodied manifestation of the perspective of the Divine.

So, I'm asking you now: When you look at what's going on in the pit of your stomach, which of these two ways of being do you get carried away with the most often?"

That is how Master Jesus began His Teaching of the third chakra, located in one hand above the navel. So the third chakra, with its double nature, expresses the incarnated "I, Me, and Myself," now named Ego, and is capable of good as well as bad since it is in possession of free will.

According to Master Jesus, the human being could begin—or not—is radical extraction of the instinctive universe of animals. Therefore, the third chakra was for Him analogous to a blaze … knowing that any blaze could prove to be destructive or lifesaving. It is no coincidence that we call this area of the body the solar plexus.

The third chakra—*Manipura* in Sanskrit, and in the Kabbalistic Tree of Life, left is *Nizha* and right is *Hod*—is located in the upper belly where Spleen and Pancreas are on the left side and Liver and Gallbladder on the right side, leading us to understand the double principle of this Fire.

To assimilate, digest and sort are directly related to the free will inherent to the human being.

According to Him, the malfunction of the organs governed by the third chakra was closely linked to the difficulties of the embodied personality. The choices that a human being must make in his life, the way in which he knows or does not know how to sort what comes to him, and the level of animalism that he manifests in certain situations therefore greatly condition the balance of his digestive functions.

By teaching us to empty our third chakra of its impurities, Master Jesus sought to reconcile us with the difficulties inherent in the world.

134

- Place your left hand on your left knee, palm down, while your right hand is positioned on your third chakra.

This first phase is based on the same main principles as those mentioned in the exercise devoted to the second chakra. However, the energy circuit created will be a little different insofar as the third chakra is more igneous than aquatic.

While the exercise of the second chakra was of a mainly lunar polarity, the exercise of the third chakra associates the moon with the sun: the image of a lunar crescent always present in our hand and our knee (left for men, right for women) will indeed be in contact with our solar plexus. This position illustrates in its own way the double aspect that the Master taught us on the third chakra, meaning the sun and its reflection, the moon.

Christ attached great importance to living the first phase of the exercise fully. He recommended that we took time in order to properly perceive the energy flow which was established in our body relative to our posture, and to capture any images or sensations that crossed us.

- With a breath in, visualize that same white sun that descended from your back to the base of your body. Move it to your third plexus and let it sit, shining, for a few seconds.

Master Jesus urged us not to lose sight of the fact that this little white sun was emanating from our higher consciousness. Our approach was based, above all, on help requested from our deepest dimension, constantly connected to the Divine.

It should be understood that without this connection with Above, the awakening and cleaning of Below, initiated by the whole exercise, only becomes a small discipline of visualization and breathing deprived of any real effects. Everything is in the orientation of the consciousness and not in the strict exercise itself.

- Then exhale powerfully, always through your nose, with a sharp blow while trying to perceive a total expansion of your aura.

This phase of the exercise is essential. When practiced correctly, one realizes that the movement of expelling air is controlled by a discharge of energy coming from the whole region of the third chakra.

In fact, it is not just the lungs that empty themselves. On the subtle planes, it is the whole sphere of organs linked to the functions of assimilation and digestion which expels from it what is called "miasmas" of used energy. These miasmas are the basic materials by which toxic cellular memories and instinctual reflexes are built and encysted. They are also the anchor point for shaped thoughts linked to the emotional universe.

As for the movement of projection of the aura which accompanies the energetic discharge emanating from the third chakra, one easily understands that it allows an evacuation of the miasmas in question out of the subtle organism.

The nasal cavities occupy a very important place here. When the dryly exploded air passes through them, they play the role of a filter which neutralizes the toxic micro-memories of what is expelled.

One has the impression that it is the lungs which get rid of used gases but, in reality, it is all the emotional or astral dimension of the being which undertakes to clean itself of its slag. Christ described this slag to us as *"invisible dust similar to a slow-acting poison."*

The state of mind with which we expel the toxins from our body through the filter of the nasal cavity was for Him one of the main components of the practice. This state of mind was the ultimate guarantee of its effectiveness.

It was not conceivable to release any kind of subtle poison seed. Such seeds would then be capable of feeding toxic egregores in the ambient atmosphere. We therefore had to, through our thought, impregnated with Love, convert, if not neutralize, what we were projecting outside of ourselves through our nostrils and our aura.

- *The ideal scenario is repeating these inhalations/ exhalations thirty-three times. You must be very careful in this practice. When it is understood well, this should not lead to hyperventilation—that is, when it is conducted peacefully and with care. You will end this exercise by observing a long inner silence.*

Purification of the Fourth Chakra

Introduction of *The Teaching of the Fourth Chakra* *according to Master Jesus*

Let us now come to the region of Beauty, that point of strength that the Easterners call *Anahata* and the Kabbalists *Tipheret*. According to the Master, the heart chakra is the center where the ideals are conceived and also from where they are manifested physically. In other words, the fourth chakra is really the place of expression of Beauty in the universal sense and on all planes where life develops.

In the great Temple, represented by the human body, the heart chakra was for Him an immaterial zone insofar as it cannot be represented by a particular symbol. He spoke of it as a place of convergence of all energy influences and all transmutations. Internally we could represent the fourth chakra in the form of a purifying basin where we had to be submerged entirely like a flame whose calcinating aspect reinitialized our life process.

However, the heart chakra was considered a "point of consciousness" suspended between worlds and belonging to each of them in the connection of the eternal present.

The archetype of Beauty, He taught, went beyond all reference because it was the seed of the Memory of God in each of us. To penetrate precisely to the heart of a Temple, it meant rejoining the memory of the path leading to our origin. This memory, He added, shined an inner space so vast that it was impossible to imagine its limits.

For us, His teaching was not symbolic or allegoric, but a tangible reality in terms of soul and spirit. And for good reason, on a special occasion, Master Jesus allowed us to live one of those experiences that no being could erase from his memory.

We were barely ten. After asking us to sit in a circle around Him, He slowly turned around Himself in order to face each of us for a few seconds. During these privileged moments and while His eyes plunged into ours, He had placed his hand lightly on the chakra of our heart. When we happily shared what we had experienced, we were forced to note that we had all made the same inner journey.

At the precise moment when the Master touched the center of our chest, each one had the physical sensation of falling silently into a bottomless well of light, not with the feet or the head forward, but really through the heart, as if the whole of his being had been sucked by him and into him.

Personally, I still remember very precisely the immensity and the infinitude of this heart abyss. Once the first sensation of falling had passed, it suddenly seemed to me that I was rather climbing towards some unknown summit and that the streams of light which enveloped my field of vision were found a multitude of small huts. Each of them—something in me knew—contained a whole world with its wonders and pettiness, clear skies and storms. It is also the image of a hive buzzing with life, with its honeycomb throats, which imposed itself on me. It was mind-blowing in power, almost scary … but at the same time, above all, incredibly sweet and loaded with unspeakable nostalgia. It all ended almost abruptly as if coming out of an ineffable dream when I knew very well that I had not fallen asleep and never lost consciousness.

He told us first of all that we could have had a roughly similar experience at the level of each of our chakras, namely the initial feeling of falling rapidly diminished in favor of an ascension.

His precise words were about this: *"When you descend into yourself, you ascend. What we take for a fall is in fact the translation of the movement of humility which pushes us to go back to our Source .... In this case, I have helped you a little, that's all ...."*

Regarding the perception of alveoli evoking those of a beehive, He clarified that these were however specific to the center of the heart. According to Him, each of the glimpsed cells corresponded to the door of a life that we had lived or that was already germinating in us. It was essential to have a clean heart since it represented the portal of absolute access to our memory and ultimately, at the top of this memory was engraved the seal of Beauty.

- *"Is this also the place of Nostalgia?"* questioned one of us.

- *"Precisely,"* replied the Master, *"because the fire castle of Beauty is surrounded by a crown of water, which is Nostalgia ... the nostalgia of our separation from Beauty. From this feeling is born this sadness which often escorts us during the wanderings of our lives. To build a bridge over its waters and rediscover the joy of Beauty, we must have made peace with all the alveoli that partition our lives."*

A question then springs unanimously from all of us:

- *"Is there no other solution than that of unraveling the tangles of each of our lives? It is a task that seems hopeless in terms of complexity ...."*

- *"Yes, there is another ... These are the access locks to what has made them so often painful that it is up to you to blow up ... These locks are always the same. We can baptize them with a multitude of names such as selfishness, laziness, brutality, greed, pride ... But in truth, however, I will tell you that there is only one lock ... It is that of fear. By cleaning the center of our chest, it is therefore that you are going 'to attack'. Not in a belligerent way but with the solvent of tenderness."*

141

By helping us free the pathways to our fourth chakra, Master Jesus made sure that the tightness of Fear, as a global blocking force, loosened its squeeze within us. This is how the exercise He taught us took on its full value ….

- Cross your arms over your chest, right over left.

This posture is reminiscent of the traditional position of the pharaohs when they are represented with the symbols of their function: the whip and the cross. The whip, named *heka*, represents the tool for protection. The cross—in which we recognize a crook—was called *nekhekh* and symbolized justice. The Egyptian cross was a tool for guidance. United and acting simultaneously, the whip and the cross embody the attributes of the Good Shepherd, symbols of the Divine Force on Earth.

Master Jesus Himself clarified to us that they were the attributes of Osiris, Master of the Heart and Guardian of the world of the dead in Egyptian Tradition. His intention was obviously not limited to this cultural aspect. He especially wanted to make us penetrate the meaning of the symbols used by the Egyptians because these symbols, he said, concealed fundamental truths.

On the energy level, He saw the area of the heart chakra as a "splash" of light whose four rays suggest the shape of a cross. He taught us that this cross was the result of two rivers of light that meet in the center of the chest of every human being. Still, according to Him, the fact of crossing both arms along the path of these two lines of force multiplies their intensity and helps vibrationally to incarnate beyond all fear. It is important that the left arm must be placed under the right arm. Why? Mainly a symbol that the Tradition asked us to respect. A true symbol always hides an archetype upstream of it and an egregore downstream, both of which give it undeniable power.

- Sit and breathe regularly, trying to perceive (without projecting forward) a flattened spiral of pink light swirling harmoniously in the center of your chest. Its direction of rotation is clockwise. Ideally, nineteen complete rotational movements will occur, and your breathing will remain at its natural pace.

It should be understood that this spiral of pink light is not imaginary. There is a whirlwind of light at the precise center of each of our chakras. This vortex is emissive on the front of the body and receptive on the back of it. In the case of the heart chakra, the meeting point between these two "polarizations" coincides with the seed-cell[4] which follows us from life to life. Christ taught us that it was the fact of allowing ourselves to be absorbed by the clockwise movement of this luminous whirlwind that allows us to enter into relationship with our past sufferings.

Thus, letting the perception of the pink luminous spiral rise in us in this exercise aims to initiate a clearing of our suffering memories.

The Master clarified to us that the pink color was not to be associated with the fourth chakra, but it was its psychologically non-aggressive and somewhat carnal radiance that made it ideal for this exercise. On the other hand, the position of the arms crossed on the chest served to limit excessive emotional manifestations.

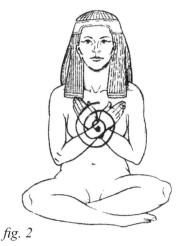

fig. 2

---

4   *See p. 23, The Great Book of Essenian & Egyptian Therapies by Daniel Meurois & Marie Johanne Croteau.*

- Then have a column of white light rise from your heart chakra to the top of your head, with a slow breath in.

The movement of this delicate luminous column upwards had to be spontaneous and experienced as "a vertical channeling of an excess of our heart." What is this excess made of? It is made of all the power of compassion that we are capable of during a spontaneous momentum.

- At the end of your breath in, once the column of light has reached above your head, let it spin and form a spiral turning clockwise. Perceive it while holding your breath briefly.

The choice of the spiral by the Master Jesus indicates to us the dynamic aspect of this exercise. If He advised us to perceive this spiral of the top of our head, only a few seconds in apnea, full lungs, it is to preserve the quality of the generated momentum without interference with the mind or an overly tense will. Here again, it is the relaxation and the joy which must prevail at the heart of the purification.

"Purification said Rabbi Jesus, does not work for mortification but for the splendor of the human being in his true dimension. To purify oneself is not to punish oneself but to be reconciled with one's original nature."

- *Ideally, this exercise will be performed four times in a row.*

Purification of the Fifth Chakra

Introduction of *The Teaching of the Fifth Chakra* according to Master Jesus

The fifth chakra—*Vishudha* in Sanskrit, and in the Kabbalistic Tree of Life, left is *Hesed* and right is *Gheboura*—is located between the two shoulders.

"These two altars—Hesed and Gheboura—of the Great Temple, Master Jesus said, serve the whirlwind of energy of the throat, the one whose initial function is to proclaim the purity of the heart. They remind us that we must learn what is right, beyond fear, in order to be able to express love in a strong and solid way."

The Easterners named *Vishudha* as a major place essential to the health of humans. The organ of communication—Larynx—a prime regulator in the human body, both physical and subtle.

Indeed, the teaching of Christ aimed at making us understand that our throat chakra regulates our whole psycho-affective sphere and the organs which are directly dependent on it, the intestines, the lungs, and the diaphragm.

"The one who speaks badly, he clarified, at first he breathes badly."

For the Master "to speak badly" was quite simply to speak with fear, fear of oneself, fear of the other, fear of life. Speaking well or badly had nothing to do with the talent of a speaker because one could express oneself very well in public but speak badly towards oneself, that is to say betraying one's own heart by suffocating it behind empty or false words.

By the misuse of the throat chakra, the human being pollutes his cellular reality by encumbering it primarily at the level of the respiratory and intestinal systems. We could add today that it weakens its thyroid with all the repercussions, not only physical, but also psychological. A person's irascibility, according to Jesus, was the mark of a disorder in the expression—or the non-expression—of fundamental suffering.

- Place your left hand on your left knee, palm up, while your right hand is positioned on your throat chakra.

In this position, it goes without saying that we generate a kind of loop of energy, a loop allowing a privileged relationship between the earth—dispenser of force by the means of the knee—and the larynx, translator of the expression of the life in the initiation of the power of sound.

"The Sound translates the overflow of a consciousness and a body. It authorizes their basic need for creation. Its expression is twofold: it illustrates the action of emptying and simultaneously that of filling. Life is an exchange, and it is for this reason that it passes through the Sound and its support— the Breath. So, I tell you, in the heart of the Word, there is the Breath." It is on these words that the Master Jesus commented on the first phase of this exercise aimed at cleaning the fifth chakra. It is important to anchor yourself well while beginning to ascend towards the upper spheres of your being.

According to Him, the force center of the throat marked the entrance of the Most Holy Place of the great human Temple. It was the area where the elements (fire, air, water, earth) of which we are made express themselves in an ethereal way. This may appear to be in conflict with the anchoring that has just been mentioned. Yet the Master did not consider Ether to be immaterial. He described it as a more tangible world capable of manifesting itself very concretely in us.

To purify the throat chakra, with its direct relation to the nadis, was equivalent to activating the key to the portal, leading to the Holy of Holies. It was to give oneself the tools to powerfully embody the perception of what is right and thereby manifest a merciful love.

- Slowly and consciously, inhale a trickle of light blue air while scraping the back of your nasal cavity with it.

Christ always associated the blue light with the Presence of the Word in Creation. He described this limpid blue as being the visible translation of Sound capable of generating forms and facts. He taught us that the intention of the Divine Principle was for us to realize that every human being is endowed with the same potential through his breath and his larynx.

The main purpose of holding our breath in full lung is to pause our consciousness for a moment. It allows a better orientation of the movement of the breathe-out in order to fully release the waste from the mental body and what has built up in the throat.

- Hold your breath (full lungs) then exhale the trickle of air in the same way, this time while visualizing a dark blue color. This will be a load of etheric waste. *Practice this respiratory movement seven times in a row to complete the "cleansing" phase of this exercise before beginning the "toning" phase.*

The dark blue with which we are going to color the stream of expelled air inside reflects the presence of mental tensions which are filtered by the nadis from the back of our nasal cavity.

The number seven, indicating the number of times to repeat the inspiration-expiration cycle, expresses, through its symbol, the cleansing and regenerating function of life.

Have we not seen that the human body takes about seven years to renew itself completely at the level of its cells?

147

- Make a buzzing sound that emanates from the back of your throat. When you approach the end of your breath, finish expelling it at once through the nose with force. *Repeat this phase five times in a row and then remain in a deep silence.*

The simple vibration in the back of the throat has the function of generating a space of mental availability and at the same time a cellular dilation of the whole area of the throat. This dilation promotes the release of painful memories. When the mouth closes and the air is finally rejected with a sharp blow through the nose, the modified prana of which it is made, releases micro ethereal particles which act as mental cement. What is rejected by the nose at the end of this exercise is therefore not an energetically polluted matter but completely neutral.

Christ's will was that we never expel from ourselves the smallest particle of life whose nature would have been etherically heavy or messy for our world.

Although we were ignorant of all notions of ecology since our material productions were in agreement with Nature, we were on the other hand well informed of the existence of psychic pollution and their impact on the human balance, right down to a cellular level.

Cleaning our fifth chakra was therefore taught to us by the Master Jesus as a gesture as basic as the one which pushes us today to brush our teeth regularly.

Purification of the Sixth Chakra

Introduction of *The Teaching of the Sixth Chakra* *according to Master Jesus*

The sixth chakra—*Ajna* in Sanskrit, and in the Kabbalistic Tree of Life, left is *Hochmah* and right is *Binah*—is located respectively to the left and right of the head.

Binah and *Hochmah*, these two sephiroth, radiate and converge in the center of the skull in a unique point. This precise point, located at the base of the brain just below the hypothalamus, is called the pituitary gland. *Binah* and *Hochmah* were described by Christ as two major elements of "a central altar supported by two pillars." The hypophysis is made up of two lobes. How do we not recognize *Binah* and *Hochmah* united to form a unique energy entity known as *Ajna*?

The fact that *Ajna* is also called "third eye" should not surprise us. A little in-depth attention paid to our constitution teaches us that the two lobes of the pituitary gland are in anatomical relation with the optic chiasm, a term which designates—behind our forehead—the zone of crossing of the optic nerves. This point of convergence of right and left vision speaks for itself.

In addition, the hypophysis actually acts as a conductor towards the endocrine glands, which allows us to deduce that the pituitary gland regulates the functioning of a large part of our chakras. What could be more logical that it is considered as the Eye of the Sage, the eye of the One who unites all aspects of Intelligence? The third eye energetically translates information from our higher consciousness to relay it to our subtle organism.

"The Sage looks at the soul behind the mask of the face, the spirit behind the smile of the soul and the Divine behind the light of the spirit."

- After putting your hands together for a few moments, bring your right hand to the root of your nose, between your two eyebrows.

After closing your eyes, calling silence and quietness in you, join your hands together as a prayer. According to the Master Jesus, the attitude of the prayer generates a kind of smoothing and rebalancing of the aura.

- Using rapid movements with your right forefinger, tap your frontal chakra with the flat of your fingernail twelve times. This will create a feeling of pressure on the area.

The repeated dry snapping of the flat of your fingernail directly on the zone of the frontal chakra must create a real stimulation there so it is very noticeable on the skin. This precise region is of great sensitivity.

The Master taught us that the whole circumscribed zone of the sixth chakra on this frontal zone is extraordinarily irrigated by a very complex network of very small nadis which extend like a myriad of silver threads between the dermis of the pituitary gland. This region is rich in vital energy which led Him to speak of the third eye as a center bathed in a luminous moon-colored liquid.

According to the Christ, by this gesture, we knocked in a way on the door of our soul, as if to "awaken" certain aspects inviting her to take a leap in matter where her extension goes skin deep. In fact, He wanted this harmless little gesture to be executed not in a mechanical way, but with a sacred intent. Our dry snaps of the flat fingernail must be, in their essence, like the gesture of a priest who calls for internal listening by ringing a bell.

Master Jesus was actually asking us to project our consciousness into the center of our skull, just as today we can project our gazes and calls to what is called the eardrum of a church.

By resonating and stimulating this zone, according to Him, the Intelligence of the Sage managed to set himself in motion in order to act as a pathfinder.

- Slowly inhale as you try to feel this inhalation moving through the frontal chakra, like you're trying to fill an air pocket behind it. Repeat this inhalation a dozen times.

Breathing here takes place through the nose. What Christ wanted was for us to experience from within, through the channel of the sixth chakra, in order to expand it psychically. According to His teaching, the dilation—well controlled—of a chakra is always a key factor for its purification as well as that of the nadis which converge towards it. In fact, the wider a canal, the less waste of all kinds will clump together and stagnate.

This comparison may seem prosaic, but we must not forget that a chakra is analogous to a light well in the form of a spiral. This spiral penetrates the body from behind and comes out from the front. What makes the deployment diameter of such a spiral? It is quite simply the quality of the being or, in other words, the alchemy which operates between the clearness and the force which the soul achieves to manifest ... even if the physical body under which she hides expresses suffering. In my memories, I can testify that I heard the Master affirm that He captured the clearness of a soul by rushing in entirely, for a very short time, between the two eyebrows, *"where the history of her wisdom and her strength are, He said, are legible at all times."*

When we replied, it seemed contradictory to the way He had spoken of the heart before. He then specified this:

151

"The heart is the door to memories then the key to Memory. It is through it that the beauty of Love is manifested, it is also through this door you remain in eternal learning since it is forever perfectible. When looking at the center of your forehead, your third eye serves to guide this beauty and the power that flows from it. Its mission is to teach you to lead them with discernment. To see through this eye is to breathe through it. It is to capture the balances and the imbalances in order to unify the lessons. It is to sneak up to the altar where the Father begins to be truly audible in the finality of His intentions .... In truth, your third eye is the lamp of your being. If your sixth chakra is in good condition, your whole being will brighten up. If not, then your being remains in the darkness of ignorance."

In the respiratory phase of the purification of the sixth chakra, the level of consciousness and love is essential for the prana to irrigate the center of our skull.

- Be cross-eyed internally without forcing it, but enough to create a feeling of pressure between your eyes. In the meantime, repeat the syllable "ta" loudly until you reach saturation (preferably no longer than one minute).

The action of converging the eyes at a single point located between the eyebrows automatically solicits the optic nerves and therefore the zone of the *optic chiasm* which, I recall, is in close energy relation with the pituitary gland.

Squinting can cause—behind our closed eyelids and in the center of our skull—a number of luminous halos and even geometric figures. These manifestations are the witnesses of the level of clearness of our inner being. The most classic shapes that appear on our interior screen are the golden ring, the blue disc, or the five-pointed star.[5]

Regarding the sound "ta," repeated loudly until you reach saturation, Rabbi Jesus explained to us that in reality we were

---

5   *See pgs. 106-107.*

pronouncing TAT by the simple effect of repeating TA. From there, He immediately came to tell us the reason for choosing this syllable. His teaching led Him to evoke certain prayers that He had repeated at length during His journey in what He sometimes called "the land of high snows."[6] He spoke to us briefly about the sacredness of the Sanskrit language which He had to practice and of the mantra TAT TVAM ASI which He pronounced thousands and thousands of times during intense periods of solitary retreat.

This mantra, He taught us, means "You are That" knowing that "THAT" represents the sound TAT. In the context of this statement, we were to understand that "THAT" means Ultimate Reality, that is, Divinity beyond what we can conceive of.

According to the Master, the TAT vibration—that of Ultimate Reality—while we stimulated our inner gaze, had the capacity to generate a purifying and unifying wave of which we had no idea of its power. The ideal was therefore to immerse ourselves completely in the ocean of peace that was gradually emerging from the deployment of this vibration.

However, once again and more than ever, we were told not to commit abuses in this practice. We had to move forward in it smoothly without personal challenges in order to harmoniously connect with the Ultimate Reality, of which the sixth chakra is constantly the translator.

---

6   *The Secret Life of Jeshua; According to the Memory of Time by Daniel Meurois.*

Purification of the Seventh Chakra

Introduction of *The Teaching of the Seventh Chakra* according to Master Jesus

The seventh chakra—*Sahasrara* in Sanskrit and *Kheter* in the Kabbalistic Tree of Life—is located at the top of our skull.

The Master compares the seventh chakra to the fontanel. In fact, this membrane located at the top of the human skull and which allows, in infants, the growth of the encephalon, corresponds precisely to the radiation of the seventh chakra. The Essenians asserted that if our soul was embodied by this point, it should also seek to leave from this same point. This knowledge joins all the great Traditions speaking of the unfolding of *the lotus with a thousand petals*.

However, Christ went further by teaching us that, when the consciousness enters the body which it is about to inhabit, it does so by descending along a kind of thin conduit of light which corresponds to the heart—or the pistil—of this lotus, all the petals of which are then closed. According to his words, this conduit can be compared to a well which descends in the depths of the being to the first chakra. Such a descent is carried out by this subtle channel which we call *Sushumma* and which serves as the central axis of the two great nadis that are *Ida* and *Pingala*.[7]

---

7   *See p. 31 The Great Book of the Essenian and Egyptian Therapies by Daniel Meurois and Marie Johanne Croteau.*

Finally, Master Jesus added that when the seventh chakra succeeds in unfolding after a very large number of lifetimes, this well expands to become a fountain of light. The energy that inhabits it manages to completely fulfill its role by descending to the heart of the first chakra and to unite with the kundalini force. Then this united flow of light ascends by joining with the *Ida* and *Pingala* currents to form a triple fire. This Triple Fire will flow freely along the spine and fluidize all the chakras by blooming in a jet of light at the exact top of the head.

- Place both hands on your knees, palms up.

- Strive to perceive the presence of a white sun above your head. This sun will drop, one after another, seven droplets of gold onto your seventh chakra. Feel these seven droplets making contact on the top of your head.

- At your own pace, practice a few long breaths in and out.

- Visualize a kind of waterfall and the touch of the seven droplets on your head.

- At your own pace again, practice a few more long breaths in and out.

- Return to your perception of the droplets one last time.

- Take some time for inner silence, and then emit a long, deep buzzing sound from the back of your throat (or the traditional **Om** if you prefer).

Purification of the Eighth Chakra

Introduction of *The Teaching of the Eighth Chakra* according to Master Jesus

- *Before beginning the eighth phase of this long practice, it will be helpful to refer to paragraph 5 of Chapter 3 of this book (p. 33-34).*

"Spirit who lives in us ignores sleep. Its radiance is felt in perpetual action at the zenith of our consciousness. Even if you think you have reached the highest point of your soul, Spirit is there to dissuade you and encourage you to climb a little higher. This is exactly what your eighth chakra teaches you, the one that holds like a flaming disc, half gold, half silver, just above your head. This disc is white like a lily with the pistil of gold. The Masters of the Past named the eighth chakra Tekla."

The role of the eighth chakra—The Great Mind—is precisely to let out of its own radiance, loving golden drops so that they gradually permeate all the levels of intelligence of our being. Its "extra corporeality" protects our eighth chakra from the pollution from which our other subtle centers regularly suffer. *Tekla* is not connected with any circuit of nadis and therefore cannot be reached by the energy slags which a number of thought forms and emotional reactions induce.

157

For Him, this exercise was one of the most beautiful that can be experienced because it was equivalent to entering into a deep relationship with the Source.

- With both hands on your knees, palms up, observe a long silence while striving in the heart of this silence to perceive the sound of prana in you (a kind of hissing in the center of your head).

- Now try to perceive yourself about one meter (or 40 inches) "in the air" above your seventh chakra, almost like the location of a showerhead.

- When this mental image is created in your inner space and you manage to "look at yourself from Above," visualize droplets of gold gently falling from the top of your head—the center of your consciousness—down through your entire body.

- Finish this exercise with a long silence with both of your arms crossed at your chest, right over left.

Also By

Sacred Worlds Publishing
www.sacredworldspublishing.com

Our books reveal timeless wisdom to awaken
and empower the soul.

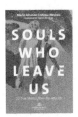

Souls Who Leave Us
12 True Stories from the Afterlife
A testimonial book, rich in information and immense compassion.

The Great Book of Essenian & Egyptian Therapies
A must read for all body workers
looking to deepen and expand their practice.

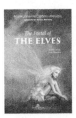

The Portal of the Elves
Memories from Elsewhere
A true tale of harmony and freedom
between lifetimes and realms.

Printed in Great Britain
by Amazon

42175063R00101